Protection of the Skin
against Ultraviolet Radiations

Éditions John Libbey Eurotext
127, avenue de la République
92120 Montrouge, France
Tél. : 01 46 73 06 60

John Libbey and Compagny Ltd
13, Smiths Yard, Summerley Street
London SW18 4HR, England
Tél. : 1 947 27 77

John Libbey CIC
Via L. Spallanzani, 11
00161 Rome, Italy
Tel. : 06 862 289

© John Libbey Eurotext, 1998, Paris
ISBN 2-7420-0246-4

Il est interdit de reproduire intégralement ou partiellement le présent ouvrage sans autorisation de l'éditeur ou du Centre Français d'Exploitation du Droit de Copie, 20, rue des Grands-Augustins, 75006 Paris.

Protection of the Skin against Ultraviolet Radiations

edited by
André Rougier
Hervé Schaefer

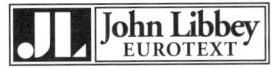

Since 1995, Dr. André Rougier is Scientific Manager of La Roche-Posay Pharmaceutical Laboratories. Between 1981 and 1989, he focused his research interest in skin permeability, barrier function and skin pharmacokinetics and published over 40 scientific papers and contributed to numerous textbooks in the field. Between 1989 and 1995 he successively had in charge the Department of Toxicology and the Research Group on Skin and Systemic Safety at the Basic Research Center of l'Oréal. During this period he centered his activities in the research and development of alternative methods to replace animal testing in toxicology. In this area of research, he published around 50 papers.

Since 1995, André Rougier took particular interest in photo-dermatology and photo-protection area in which he published over 30 scientific papers.

In his carrier, André Rougier contributed to numerous textbooks in the field of skin biology ans skin pharmacology.

André Rougier is Member of the American Academy of Dermatology, the Society for Investigative Dermatology, the American Academy of Sciences, the European Academy of Dermatology and Venereology, the International Society of Contact Dermatitis, the American Association of Pharmaceutical Scientists, the Tissue Culture Association, the European Culture Society, the International Society of Cosmetic Chemists.

In 1985 and 1986 he was awarded by the American Society of Cosmetic Chemists for his contribution in skin research.

André Rougier received his Ph. D. from the University of Paris in 1975.

*
* **

Professor Hans Schaefer is scientific director at l'Oréal, Clichy/France. He received his Ph. D. of chemisty and biochemistry at the University of Bonn in Germany. From 1965 to 1969 he was head of the dermatology laboratory at Thomac, a pharmaceutical company in Biberach/ Germany. In 1969 he joined the Free University of Berlin and became head of the research laboratory of the dermatology department of the Rudolf Virchow Hospital. In 1972 he was appointed as professor for biochemistry in dermatology.

In 1978-1979 he was invited as visiting professor to the dermatology department of the Medical School at the Stanford University.

In 1979 he joined the cosmetics compagny l'Oréal as director of the biology department. At the same time he founded the CIRD (Centre International des Recherches Dermatologiques) in Sophia Antipolis in the South of France, which he directed until 1992 and which has now about 200 collaborators.

He cochaired the 1997 Gordon Conference on the "Barrier function of mammalian skin" and will chair this conference in 1999.

His main research interests are in skin physiology, in skin pharmacology and in particular in percutaneous absorption and the skin barrier, on which subjects he has initiated and conducted numerous research projects and written or edited several books.

... « *Predicting chronic effects of UV based only on acute exposures is completely misleading. Even small amounts of UVA received chronically is damaging* »...

Albert Kligman

Contents

Are UVA rays dangerous? A. Rougier	1
Population exposure to solar UVA radiation B.L. Diffey	11
Influences of UVA in experimental photocarcinogenesis P.D. Forbes	15
Photocarcinogenesis by UVA (365-nm) radiation A. de Laat, H.J. van Kranen, J.C. van der Leun, F.R. de Gruijl	19
Does UVA exposure cause human malignant melanoma ? A.R. Young	25
UVA and oxidative stress L. Dubertret	29
In vivo **biological effects of UVA and sunscreen efficacy studies** A.M.-A. Fourtanier	33
Molecular aspects of photoaging J. Uitto, D.B. Brown, F.P. Gasparro, E.F. Bernstein	37
Effects of repeated suberythemal doses of UVA in human skin S. Seité, D. Moyal, S. Richard, J. de Rigal, J.-L. Lévêque, C. Hourseau, A. Fourtanier	47
Effects of repeated low doses of solar simulated UVR in human. Comparison with severe photodamaged skin S. Seité, S. Tison-Régnier, F. Christiaens, M.-P. Verdier, , P. Piquemal, C. Monstatier, A. Fourtanier	59
Expression of DNA-damage and stress proteins by UVA irradiation of human skin *in vivo* Lee A. Applegate, C. Scaletta, A. Fourtanier, R.E. Mascotto, S. Seité, E. Frenk	73
Mechanisms of UV-induced immunosuppression. Link between UV-induced tolerance and apoptosis T. Schwarz	83
Dose-responses for UV-induced suppression of various immune responses T. Kim, S.E. Ullrich, M.L. Kripke	87
UV-induced immunosuppression. The critical role of wavelength B. Jan Vermeer, M. Wintzen, F.H.J. Class, A.A. Schothorst, H.M.H. Hurks	89
Effects of UVA light on the immune system. A settled issue? T. Schwarz	93
Ultraviolet A radiation-induced immunomodulation: molecular and photobiological mechanisms J. Krutmann	97
UVA1 radiation-induced immunomodulatory and gene regulatory effects in human keratinocytes J. Krutmann	103
Immunomodulation by UV light: role of neuropeptides T.A. Luger	107
Relevance of photo-immunosuppression for viral infections (*i.e.* human papillomavirus) B.J. Vermeer, J.N. Bouwes Bavinck	111

Immunomodulation induced by psoralen plus ultraviolet A radiation
F. Aubin, Ph. Humbert 115

Recent advances in sun protection
H. Schaefer, D. Moyal, A. Fourtanier 119

Persistent pigment darkening as a method for the UVA protection assessment of sunscreens
A. Chardon, D. Moyal, C. Hourseau 131

Suncare product photostability: a key parameter for a more realistic *in vitro* efficacy evaluation.
Part I: *in vitro* efficacy assessment
B.L. Diffey, R.P. Stokes, S. Forestier, C. Mazilier, A. Richard, A. Rougier 137

Suncare product photostability: a key parameter for a more realistic *in vitro* efficacy evaluation.
Part II: chromatographic analysis
S. Forestier, C. Mazilier, A. Richard, A. Rougier 143

Which kind of protection a broad absorption UVA sunscreen provide?
A. Fourtanier, C. Cohen, A. Guéniche, R. Ley, D. Moyal, S. Seité 149

Effects of repetitive doses of solar simulated UVR in human skin. Protection by a daily use cream
S. Seité, P. Piquemal, C. Montastier, S. Tison-Regnier, A. Guéniche,
F. Chistiaens, A. Fourtanier 159

Disparate effects of photoprotection on ultraviolet radiation-induced immunosuppression
P.R. Bergstresser 167

Immunosuppression induced by chronic ultraviolet irradiation in humans and its prevention by sunscreens
D. Moyal 171

Photoprotection and photo-immunosuppression in man
L. Meunier 179

Influence of high protective sunscreens on the photoisomerization of urocanic acid in human skin
P. Krien, D. Moyal, A. Rougier 183

The use of a reconstructed epidermis in the evaluation of protective effect of sunscreens against lipoperoxidation induced by UVA
C. Cohen, R. Roguet, M. Cottin, M.H. Grandidier, E. Popovic, J. Leclaire, A. Rougier ... 189

The use of a reconstructed epidermis in the evaluation of protective effect of sunscreens against chemical phototoxicity induced by UVA
C. Cohen, R. Roguet, M. Cottin, C. Olive, J. Leclaire, A. Rougier 195

Prevention of solar urticaria using a broadspectrum sunscreen and determination of a solar urticaria protection factor (SUPF)
J.L. Peyron, N. Raison-Peyron, J. Meynadier, D. Moyal, A. Rougier, C. Hourseau 201

Pretreatment of human skin with a sunscreen or dihydroxy-acetone (DHA) prevents photoprovocation-induced polymorphous light eruption (PLE) and keratinocyte (KC) ICAM-1 expression
H. Stege, C. Ahrens, C. Billmann-Eberwein, T. Ruzicka, A. Richard, A. Rougier,
J. Krutmann 207

List of contributors

Ahrens C., Department of Dermatology, University of Dusseldorf, Germany.

Applegate L.A., Department of Dermatology, Laboratory of Photobiology, University Hospital-CHUV BT-04-423, CH-1011 Lausanne, Switzerland.

Aubin F., Department of Dermatology, University Hospital, Besançon, France.

Bergstresser P.R., Department of Dermatology, UT Southwestern Medical Center, Dallas, Texas, USA.

Bernstein E.F., Departments of Dermatology and Cutaneous Biology, and Biochemistry and Molecular Pharmacology, Jefferson Medical College, and the Jefferson Institute of Molecular Medicine, Thomas Jefferson University, 233 South 10th Street, Suite 450, Philadelphia, Pennsylvania, 19107, USA.

Billmann-Eberwein C., Department of Dermatology, University of Dusseldorf, Germany.

Bouwes Bavinck J.N., Department of Dermatology, Leiden University Medical Center, PO Box 9600, 2300 RC Leiden, The Netherlands.

Brown D.B., Departments of Dermatology and Cutaneous Biology, and Biochemistry and Molecular Pharmacology, Jefferson Medical College, and the Jefferson Institute of Molecular Medicine, Thomas Jefferson University, 233 South 10th Street, Suite 450, Philadelphia, Pennsylvania, 19107, USA.

Chardon A., L'Oréal, Clichy, France.

Christiaens F., Life Sciences, L'Oréal Advanced Research Laboratories, Clichy, France.

Class F.H.J., Immunohematology and Blood Bank, University Medical Center Leiden, Leiden, The Netherlands.

Cohen C., Life Sciences, L'Oréal Advanced Research Laboratories, Aulnay-sous-Bois, France.

Cottin M., Life Sciences, L'Oréal Advanced Research Laboratories, Aulnay-sous-Bois, France.

Diffey B., Medical Physics Department, General Hospital, Newcastle NE4 6BE, UK.

Dubertret L., Institut de Recherche sur la Peau, Hôpital Saint-Louis, 1, avenue Claude-Vellefaux, F-75475, Paris Cedex 10, France.

Forbes P.D., Argus Research Laboratories, Inc., Genzyme Transgenics Corp., 905 Sheehy Drive, Horsham, PA 19044, USA.

Forestier S., L'Oréal Applied Research and Development, Clichy, France.

Fourtanier A.M.-A., L'Oréal, Centre de Recherche Charles-Zviak, 90, rue du Général-Roguet, 92583 Clichy Cedex, France.

Frenk E., Department of Dermatology, Laboratory of Photobiology, University Hospital-CHUV BT-04-423, CH-1011 Lausanne, Switzerland.

Gasparro F.P., Departments of Dermatology and Cutaneous Biology, and Biochemistry and Molecular Pharmacology, Jefferson Medical College, and the Jefferson Institute of Molecular Medicine, Thomas Jefferson University, 233 South 10th Street, Suite 450. Philadelphia, Pennsylvania, 19107, USA.

Grandidier M.H., Life Sciences, L'Oréal Advanced Research Laboratories, Aulnay-sous-Bois, France.

Gruijl de F.R., Dermatology, University Hospital AZU, Utrecht, The Netherlands.

Guéniche A., Life Sciences, L'Oréal Advanced Research Laboratories, Clichy, France.

Hourseau C., L'Oréal, Centre Eugène-Schueller, 92117 Clichy Cedex, France.

Humbert Ph., Department of Dermatology, University Hospital, Besançon, France.

Hurks H.M.H., Department of Dermatology, University Hospital Leiden, PO Box 9600, 2300 RC, Leiden, The Netherlands.

Kim T., Department of Immunology, The University of Texas, MD Anderson Cancer Center, Houston, TX, USA.

Krien P., Life Sciences, L'Oréal Advanced Research Laboratories, Clichy, France.

Krutmann J., Department of Dermatology. Heinrich-Heine-University, Moorenstrasse 5, D-40225 Düsseldorf, Germany.

Kripke M.L., Department of Immunology, The University of Texas, M.D. Anderson Cancer Center, Houston, TX, USA.

Laat de A., Dermatology, University Hospital AZU, Utrecht, The Netherlands.

Leclaire J., Life Sciences, L'Oréal Advanced Research Laboratories, Aulnay-sous-Bois, France.

Lévêque J.-L., L'Oréal, Centre de Recherche Charles-Zviak, 90, rue du Général-Roguet, 92583 Clichy Cedex, France.

Ley R., The Lovelace Institutes, Albuquerque, USA.

Luger T.A., Ludwig Boltzmann Insitute for Cell Biology and Immunobiology of the Skin, Department of Dermatology, University of Münster, Münster, Germany.

Mascotto R.E., L'Oréal, Centre de Recherche Charles-Zviak, 90, rue du Général-Roguet, 92583 Clichy Cedex, France.

Mazilier C., L'Oréal Applied Research and Development, Clichy, France.

Meunier L., Department of Dermatology-Allergology-Photobiology, Saint-Éloi Hospital, University of Montpellier, Montpellier, France.

Meynardier J., Department of Dermatology, Saint-Éloi Hospital, Montpellier, France.

Montastier C., L'Oréal, Applied Research and Development, Chevilly-Larue, France.

Moyal D., L'Oréal, Centre Eugène-Schueller, 92117 Clichy Cedex, France.

Olive C., Life Sciences, L'Oréal Advanced Research Laboratories, Aulnay-sous-Bois, France.

Peyron J.L., Department of Dermatology, Saint-Éloi Hospital, Montpellier, France.

Piquemal P., L'Oréal, Applied Research and Development, Chevilly-Larue, France.

Popovic E., Life Sciences, L'Oréal Advanced Research Laboratories, Aulnay-sous-Bois, France.

Raison-Peyron N., Department of Dermatology, Saint-Éloi Hospital, Montpellier, France.

Richard A. La Roche-Posay Pharmaceutical Laboratories, 86270 La Roche-Posay, France.

Richard S., L'Oréal, Centre de Recherche Charles-Zviak, 90, rue du Général-Roguet, 92583 Clichy Cedex, France.

Rigal de J., L'Oréal, 1, avenue Eugène-Schueller, 93601 Aulnay-sous-Bois Cedex, France.

Roguet R., Life Sciences, L'Oréal Advanced Research Laboratories, Aulnay-sous-Bois, France.

Rougier A., La Roche-Posay Pharmaceutical Laboratories, 11, avenue Dubonnet, Courbevoie, France.

Ruzicka T., Department of Dermatology, University of Dusseldorf, Germany.

Scaletta C., Department of Dermatology, Laboratory of Photobiology, University Hospital-CHUV BT-04-423, CH-1011 Lausanne, Switzerland.

Schaefer H., L'Oréal Research, Clichy, France.

Schothorst A.A., Department of Dermatology, University Hospital Leiden, P.O. Box 9600, 2300 RC. Leiden, The Netherlands.

Schwarz T., Departement of Dermatology, University of Münster, Von Esmarch Strasse 56, D-48149 Münster, Germany.

Seité S., L'Oréal, Centre de Recherche Charles-Zviak, 90, rue du Général-Roguet, 92583 Clichy Cedex, France.

Stege H., Department of Dermatology, University of Dusseldorf, Germany.

Stokes R.P., Dryburn Hospital, Durham, United Kingdom.

Tison-Regnier S., L'Oréal, Centre de Recherche Charles-Zviak, 90, rue du Général-Roguet, 92583 Clichy Cedex, France.

Uitto J., Departments of Dermatology and Cutaneous Biology, and Biochemistry and Molecular Pharmacology, Jefferson Medical College, and the Jefferson Institute of Molecular Medicine, Thomas Jefferson University, 233 South 10th Street, Suite 450, Philadelphia, Pennsylvania, 19107, USA.

Ullrich S.E., Department of Immunology, The University of Texas, MD Anderson Cancer Center, Houston, TX, USA.

van Kranen H.J., Dermatology, University Hospital AZU, Utrecht, The Netherlands.

van der Leun J.C., Dermatology, University Hospital AZU, Utrecht, The Netherlands.

Verdier M.-P., L'Oréal, Centre de Recherche Charles-Zviak, 90, rue du Général-Roguet, 92583 Clichy Cedex, France.

Vermeer B.J., Department of Dermatology, University Hospital Leiden, PO Box 9600, 2300 RC Leiden, The Netherlands.

Wintzen M., Department of Dermatology, University Hospital Leiden, PO Box 9600, 2300 RC Leiden, The Netherlands.

Young A.R., UMDS, Department of Dermatology, St Thomas' Hospital, London, UK.

Are UVA rays dangerous?

André Rougier

A. Rougier: La Roche-Posay Pharmaceutical Laboratories, Courbevoie, France.

Since ultraviolet B rays (UVB, 290-320 nm) have 1,000 times the energy of ultraviolet A rays (UVA, 320-400 nm), they have long been considered to be responsible for the development of most human photodermatoses. The increased use of UVA sources over the last decade in the treatment of certain dermatoses and in artificial tanning has led photobiologists and photodermatologists to speculate about the cutaneous damage likely to be caused by this kind of radiation in the course of our everyday life rather than in exceptional exposure conditions.

The proportion of UVA rays emitted by the sun and reaching the Earth's surface is ten times that of UVB rays. Unlike UVB rays, UVA rays are not attenuated by the ozone layer surrounding our planet. They pass through clouds and glass, and are emitted at a constant rate throughout the day from sunrise to sunset. Finally, while 90% of UVB radiation is blocked by the stratum corneum, over 50% of the UVA radiation received is capable of penetrating deep into the cutaneous structures as far as the papillary and reticular derma.

UVA and photoaging

It has long been thought that the majority of human photolesions were due to UVB rays [1]. Unlike UVB rays, UVA rays do not trigger the well-known alarm signal of sunburn. Unless we are careful, therefore, UVA rays can cause greater cumulative changes than UVB rays [2], including epidermal hyperplasia with the presence of photodyskeratosic cells (a sign of damages to the DNA) [3-5], reduction of the number of Langerhans cells [6-8], latent inflammation of the dermis with vascular and collagen damage [9, 10] and lymphocytic infiltration [11], splitting of the lamina densa [4], disorganization of the elastic fibre network and expression of lysozyme [12] leading to changes in the biomechanical properties of the skin [13].

Moreover, there is a mounting quantity of evidence that large doses of UVA rays can produce changes similar to those caused by long-term exposure to solar radiation [14]. These observations have stimulated interest not only in the clinical effects but also in the mechanisms involved in the appearance of lesions due to UVA rays at cellular and molecular levels [15]. The involvement of mechanisms such as activated states of oxygen generated after UVA irradiation have been given particular attention [16].

A dose of the order of 20 joules/cm^2 on the skin for 5 weeks, which corresponds with the daily suberythemal UVA dose we are likely to receive daily in our latitudes, can produce all the effects referred to above and, in the long term, cause clinical signs of actinic aging [5]. These signs include the premature formation of wrinkles and lines which give the skin a wizened, often blotchy appearance, dotted with blemishes resulting in actinic keratosis [17-19]. More recently, it has been shown that 8 exposures to only 0.5 MED of UVA rays is enough to produce the same results [20].

Of course, this does not mean that UVA rays are the sole cause of the phenomena observed in the process of actinic aging. Many studies show that UVB rays play a very substantial role in these phenomena. However, while the part played by UVB rays in the expression of various extracellular matrix genes (particularly elastin) is very significant, the presence of UVA rays accelerates and aggravates these effects [21].

UVA rays and cancer

Having a suntan has long been synonymous with beauty, good health and dynamism in our culture. This has given rise to the development and uncontrolled use of high-pressure UVA sources. Moreover, exposures to solar radiation have become increasingly longer over the years, helped by the use of sun blocks which are often efficient against UVB but not necessarily UVA rays. Unfortunately, in addition to cutaneous damage leading to accelerated aging, UVA rays can cause even more serious cellular lesions in the long term and do so in a much more insidious way than UVB rays.

It has now been clearly established that, at the cellular level, and via various chromophores capable of absorbing their energy, UVA rays generate radicals which can cause damage to membranous lipids [22, 23] and proteins, and lead to the destruction of DNA [24]. This produces far-reaching alterations leading to changes in cell nutrition, receptivity to growth factors [25] and effectiveness of the cutaneous immune system. It is worth noting that the scope of action of the production of activated states of oxygen at the cutaneous level has been measured. The results have shown that short wavelength UVA rays (320-340 nm) appear to be more active in this area than UVB rays [26].

The final stage of the deleterious effects of UV rays is cell mutation. Here too, the active contribution of UVA rays becomes increasingly clear as our knowledge advances. For example, recent studies [12, 27] have shown that doses as small as 1-2 MED and even repeated suberythemal does of UVA can lead to DNA damage (pyrimidine dimers, sunburn cells, p53 induction, ferritin expression in the basal and suprabasal regions of the epidermis, and tenasein expression in the extracellular matrix of the dermis. All these precocious events in the cancerization process are present after irradiation purely with UVA rays.

From the clinical viewpoint, numerous animal studies have shown clearly that UVA rays on their own can cause the development of tumours [28-31]. Furthermore, combined UVA and UVB irradiation has been shown to have synergistic effects on carcinogenesis [32]. *A priori*, there is no reason why this should not be the same in humans. A question of even greater clinical interest has been raised recently with growing acuity: are UVA wavelength rays also capable of causing the development of malignant melanomas [33]?

Malignant melanomas are among the most worrying health problems of today in the developed countries, representing 3% of cutaneous cancers and some 2% of all cancers. They account for 1% of deaths due to cancer, and thus their prognosis is extremely severe. Young individuals of phototypes I and II are the most directly concerned. However, available epidemiological studies do not allow accurate identification of the guilty solar radiation wavelengths. Moreover, there are no really satisfactory animal models. However, recent studies carried out using Xiphophorus, a species of fish particularly susceptible to the development of melanomas [33], have shown the role of UVA rays to be significant in comparison with UVB rays. This importance of UVA radiation could be due to the generation of procarcinogenic photoproducts from eumelanin and particularly from pheomelanin. Even if there is a world of difference between a fish and a human being, it would be unreasonable to ignore this type of result. Thus a recent controlled study [34] showed that the use of sunscreen products effective solely in the UVB range could be a risk factor for melanoma development. This would apply equally in the case of sunlamp users [35].

UVA rays and the immune system

While studying the cancerization process, it is entirely logical to think that this process could be facilitated by immune system deficiencies [36, 37]. This is why numerous works have been devoted to the immunosuppressant effects of UV radiation in recent years.

While the procarcinogenic activity of ultraviolet radiation has been known for a century, it was realised only very recently that exposing the skin to the sun leads to far-reaching changes in the immune response.

Experiments carried out primarily on the naked mouse [38, 39] have, in particular, shown the delayed contact hypersensitization reaction to a powerful allergenic to be suppressed by UV irradiation, whether at the time of contact with the allergenic (induction) or at the time of challenge. Moreover, this immunosuppression can be induced by UV radiation remote from the allergen administration site, showing that solar radiation is capable of causing not only a local but also a general immunosuppressant effect.

It is now clearly established that these changes can contribute significantly to the development of cutaneous cancers and facilitate the installation of infectious diseases, opening up a new and very important field of research: photoimmunology.

It is difficult to consider a probable involvement of UVA rays in cutaneous carcinogenesis without envisaging their action on the immune system [40, 41]. However, while there are numerous studies relating to the effects of UVB rays on the immune response and their involvement in cutaneous carcinogenesis and the exacerbation of certain infectious diseases, there are very many less studies implicating UVA rays since they are more recent, even though the fact that PUVA therapy leads to inhibition of the immune response [42, 43] has long been known.

As with UVB rays, UVA rays are capable of inducing morphological and biochemical changes in the epidermal dendritic cells, particularly the Langerhans cells, by modifying their functionality (mobility, membranal adhesion molecules) [44-47]. In contrast to UVB rays, UVA ray doses of the order of 20 J/cm^2 do not suppress the delayed hypersensitization reaction to a hapten. However, in the current state of affairs, nothing enables us to conclude that this might not be the case for larger UVA ray doses of the order of 60 J/cm^2, which represent entirely realistic daily doses in certain regions. Finally, it has been shown that volunteers subjected to pure UVA irradiation exhibited a depletion of killer lymphocytes involved in the elimination of precancerous cells.

Although the mechanisms involved in the immunological changes induced by UVA radiation are not yet well-known, it is likely that they can be associated with the generation of free radicals and singulet oxygen, and also with induction in the epidermis of a trans-cis isomerization of urocanic acid [48, 49], an endogenic compound frequently incriminated in the immunosuppressant effects of UVB rays. Other factors such as functional changes in the Langerhans cells, the appearance of suppressor T lymphocytes [50] facilitating the apoptosis of Langerhans cells (which lose their antigenic presentation capacity) [51], the induction of immunosuppressive cytokins (IL 10) by certain neuropeptides such as α-MSH (Melanocyte Stimulating Hormone) [52, 53] and failures in DNA repair mechanisms (endonucleases) have been highlighted recently [54, 55]. Finally, among numerous problems induced by UV irradiation, the AP2 gene involved in various immunodependent photodermatoses could be expressed after UV irradiation via the production of certain ceramides contained in intercellular cements of the stratum corneum [56].

All the fields show clearly that the immunodepressant effects of UV radiation in general can facilitate the installation of a large number of cutaneous disorders and the occurrence of cancers. This insidious action, which can occur at low irradiation doses, shows once again, if this were needed, that caution is necessary with ultraviolet radiation and protective measures are necessary. Thus it has been shown clearly that high SPF filtration (mainly effective against UVB rays) does not suffice to protect against immunodepression, and that only those products covering the entire spectrum (UVA and UVB rays) can achieve this [57]. Very recently, the major part played by UVA rays in the process of photoimmunodepression has been confirmed incontestably. The reactivity of healthy volunteers to "Multitest Mérieux" was shown to be greatly inhibited after the irradiation of areas tested not only with a solar spectrum of UVA + UVB rays, but also after irradiation with UVA alone, irrespective of whether they are of short (UVA II, 320-340 nm) or long (UVA I, 340-400 nm) wavelengths. Equally, a series of experiments carried out in the sun, under normal conditions of use, established clearly that protection against immunodepressive effects did not correlate in any way with SPF figures (erythemal); yet again, this shows the limits of this criterion in the choice of a truly protective sunscreen product. Thus it is absolutely essential to use wide spectrum sunscreen products covering both UVA and UVB rays.

In addition to the problems associated with the risk of chronic immunosuppression caused by UVA rays, beneficial effects can be seen in certain cases. Recently it has been shown that long-wavelength UVA phototherapy (UVA I, 340-400 nm) greatly improves the condition of subjects afflicted with atopic eczema by the local expression of gamma interferon, the reduction of the keratinocytic adhesion molecule ICAM-1 and dendritic epidermic cells receptive to IgE.

UVA, exogeneous photosensitizations and photodermatoses

Besides the direct actions of UVA rays on the immune system, photosensitization reactions also occur which can be induced by skin contact with certain compounds. Exogenic photosensitizations cover two large types of clinical scenarios, phototoxicity and photoallergy. These two types of reaction may be differentiated according to their aetiology and their clinical characteristics. In general, phototoxic reactions occur more frequently than the photoallergic variety. Usually, they take the form of intense sunburn followed by hyperpigmentation, while photoallergic reactions can present eczematic, papular, vesicobulous lesions. Phototoxic reactions require contact with relatively large quantities of the product, unlike the case of photoallergic reactions, which are not dose-dependent but which require repeated contacts.

It should be noted that 70% of potential phototoxins and photoallergens are active under the influence of UVA rays [59]. The phototoxins include psoralins, porphyrins, tars, benzoyl peroxide, certain antibiotics (cyclins) and certain non-steriod anti-inflammatory substances. The photoallergens include certain perfumes, some sun filters, allergens of vegetable origin, some antibiotics, certain non-steriod anti-inflammatory substances and some neuroleptics. The most susceptible anatomical regions are, of course, those most exposed to the sun: the ears, nose, cheeks, the lower part of the nape of the neck, lateral regions of the neck, the posterior parts of the forearms and the hands.

There are several potential mechanisms. When light interacts with a photosensitizing chemical in the skin, it excites electrons in the photosensitizer, creating unstable singlet or triplet states. Compounds with resonating structures, often with alternating single and double bonds or with aromatic rings, are particularly likely to cause photosensitivity reactions [60]. Energy transfer from these compounds occurs as those unstable molecules return to their ground state. The transferred energy causes damage to cellular macromolecules and cellular components, as well as the generation of inflammatory mediators. Phototoxic reactions are classified as being oxygen-dependent or non-oxygen-dependent. In the presence of oxygen, the absorption of UVA rays by some molecules leads to the formation of radical states and singlet oxygen, which are toxic to the cells. This is the case with haematoporphyrins used in dynamic phototherapy. Other molecules can be transformed into toxic products under UVA irradiation without requiring the action of oxygen. The photoproducts can then react with other endogenic molecules such as DNA. 8 MOP functions in this way. Finally, potentially photoallergenic compounds induce a type IV cellular mediation immunological reaction during which the presence of light is required for the production of reactive photoproducts capable of attaching themselves to a protein to form an antigen which can then be presented to the Langerhans cells and, via the activation of T lymphocytes, initiate the chain of events involved in delayed contact hypersensitivity. All these photosensitivity phenomena by exogenous substances may be avoided by he use of effective full-spectrum sun block particularly covering the UVA range of wavelengths [61].

Some dermatoses can be caused by exposure to sunlight. Some of these occur frequently, such as benign summer sunburn [62, 63], actinic prurigo, melasma [64] and most erythematas [65]; other more episodic dermatoses include solar urticaria. It is now clearly established that UVA rays are strongly implicated in the aetiology of dermatoses, either alone or in synergy with UVB rays. In general, these pathologies may be prevented by the use of wide-spectrum sun protection products [66-69].

UVA and photoprotection

Bearing in mind the evidence available today, our reply to the question "are UVA rays dangerous?" is in the affirmative. Protection is required, but how?

Faced with the profusion of products currently available, it is no easy task for consumers to choose a truly effective sun protection product suited to their needs and ways of life. Obviously, consumers are unable to incorporate all the – frequently complicated – parameters required for flawless protection against the short-term and long-term effects of solar radiation. In this field, the advice of a dermatologist is of primordial importance.

A very large number of high-protection sun formulas are available on the market. As far as most consumers are concerned, the main deleterious effect of overexposure is sunburn. They are not always aware of the long-term effects which may be caused by prolonged and repeated exposure. Some manufacturers have taken advantage of this relative ignorance of the danger by highlighting high UVB protection factors as a measure of their products' photoprotective qualities. This allows them to remain silent about the mediocre UVA filtration properties of their products. Consumers, believing themselves to be fully protected, then extend their exposures and thereby receive massive doses of UVA rays, whose evil effects we have seen. Other types of products display their protection factors against both UVA and UVB rays. Unfortunately, in most cases the UVA filtration systems used are not photostable. They run the risk of degradation and becoming rapidly ineffective under the action of sunlight. Worse still, during this degradation they can give rise to the production of potentially toxic or allergenic photoproducts. The photostability of their component filtration systems must, therefore, be an important criterion of choice, which unfortunately is not always the case.

Finally, in addition to good spectral cover, the ideal sun protection product must remain effective throughout the duration of long exposure times [70].

References

1. Kaminer MS. *In Photodamage: Magnitude of the Problem.* B. Gilchrest ed., Blackwell Scientific, Cambridge, 1995; pp. 1-11.
2. Bisset DL, Hannon DP, McBride JF, Patrick LF. Photoaging of skin by UVA. In *Biological Response to Ultraviolet A radiation*, F. Urbach ed., Valdenmar Publishing Company, 1992; pp. 181-8.
3. Kligman AM, Lavker RM. Cutaneous aging: The differences between intrinsic aging and photoaging. *J Cut Aging Cosmet Dermatology* 1988; 1: 5-11.
4. Lavker RM. Structural alterations in exposed and non exposed human skin. *J Invest Dermatol* 1979; 73: 59-66.
5. Lavker RM, Gerberick GF, Veres D, Irwin CJ, Kaidley KH. Cumulative effects from repeated exposures to suberythemal doses of UVB and UVA in human skin. *J Am Acad Dermatol* 1995; 32: 53-62.
6. Gilchrest BA, Szabo G, Flynn E. Chronologic and actinically induced aging in human facial skin. *J Invest Dermatol* 1983; 80: 81-5s
7. Czernielewski JM, Masouye I, Pisani A. Effects of chronic sun exposure on human Langerhans cell densities. *Photodermatology* 1999; 5: 116-20.
8. O'Dell B, Jessen R, Becker L. Diminished immune response in sun damaged skin. *Arch Dermatol.*1980: 116.
9. Kligman L. UVA induced biochemical changes in hairless mouse skin collagen: A contrast to UVB effects. In *Biological Response to Ultraviolet A radiation*, F. Urbach ed., Valdenmar Publishing Company, 1992; pp. 209-16.
10. Young AR, Plastow RS, Harisson JA, Walker SL, Hawk LM. In *Biological Response to Ultraviolet A radiation*, F. Urbach ed., Valdenmar Publishing Company, 1992; pp. 217-24.
11. Lavker RM, Kligman AM. Chronic heliodermatitis: a morphologic evaluation of chronic actinic damage with emphasis on the role of mast cells. *J Invest Dermatol* 1988; 90: 325-30.

12. Séité S, Moyal D, Richard S, de Rigal J, Lévêque JL, Hourseau C, Fourtanier A. Effect of repeated suberythemal doses of UVA in human skin. *European J Dermatol* 1997; 7, 3: 204-9.
13. Matsuoka LY, Uitto J. In Alterations in the elastic fibers in cutaneous aging and solar elasttosis. Balin AK and AM Kligman eds., Raven press, New York 1989; pp. 141-51.
14. Kligman LH, Gebre M. Biochemical changes in hairless mouse skin collagen after chronic exposure to UVA-radiation. *Photochem Photobiol* 1991; 54: 233-7
15. Peak MJ, Peak JG. In Molecular Photobiology of UVA, F. Urbach and R.W. Gange eds., Prager, New York, 1986; pp. 42-52.
16. Pathak MA, Dalle Carbonare M. In Biological Response to Utraviolet A radiation, F Urbach ed., Valdenmar Publishing Company, 1992; pp. 189-208.
17. Gilchrest BA, Soter NA, Stoff JS, Mihm MC. The human sunburn reaction. Histologic and biochemical studies. *J Am Acad Dermatol* 1981; 5: 411-22.
18. Kligman LH, Kligman AM. In Photoaging. TB Fitzpatrick ed., McGraw Hill, New York 1986; pp. 470-5.
19. Taylor CR, Stern RS, Leyden JJ, Gilchrest BA. Photoaging/photodamage and photoprotection. *J Am Acad Dermatol* 1990; 22: 1-15.
20. Lavker RM, Gerberick GF, Veres D, Irwin CJ, Kaidley KH. Quantitative assessment of cummulative damage from repetitive exposures to suberythemogenic doses of UVA in human skin. *Photochem Photobiol* 1995; 62: 348-52.
21. Uitto J, Matsuoka L, Kornberg RL. in Elastic fibers in cutaneous elastosis. R Rudolph ed., CCV. Mosby, St Louis 1986; chap. 15.
22. Morlière P, Moysan A, Santus R, Hüppe G, Maière JC, Dubertret L. UVA-induced lipid peroxidation in cultured human fibroblasts. *Biochimica Biophysica Acta* 1991; 1084: 261-8.
23. Rougier A, Cohen C, Roguet R. Skin equivalents to measure phototoxicicity. In Dermatotoxicology Methods, FN Marzulli, HI Maibach eds., Taylor and Francis, *Bristol* 1998; pp. 337-348.
24. Sutherland BM, Hacham H, Gange RW, Sutherland JC. Pyrimidine dimers formation by UVA radiation: Implication for photoreaction. In Biological Response to Utraviolet A radiation, F Urbach ed., Valdenmar Publishing Company 1992; pp.47-58.
25. Morlière P, Moysan A, Tirache J. Action spectrum for UV-induced lipid peroxidation in cultured human skin fibroblasts. *Free Radical Biology and Medicine* 1995; 19, 3: 365-71.
26. Djavaheri-Mergny M, Mazière C, Santus R, Dubertret L, Mazière JC. Ultraviolet A decreases epidermal growth factor (EGF) processing in cultured human fibroblasts and keratinocytes: inhibition of EGF-induced diacylglycerol formation. *J Invest Dermatol* 1994; 102, 2: 192-196.
27. Applegate LA, Scaletta C, Fourtanier A, Mascotto RE, Seite S, Frenk E. Expression of DNA damage and stress proteins by UVA irradiation of human skin *in vivo. Eur J Dermatol* 1997; 7, 3: 215-9.
28. De Gruijl FR, Sterenborg HJCM, Forbes PD, Davies RE, Cole C, Kelfkens G, van Weelden H, Slaper H, van der Leun JC. Wavelenght dependence of skin cancer induction by ultraviolet irradiation of albino hairless mice. *Cancer Res* 1993; 53: 53-60.
29. Forbes PD. Relative effectiveness of UVA and UVB for photocarcinogenesis. In: The Biological Effect of UVA radiation. F. Urbach and R.W. Gange eds., Praeger Publishers, New York 1986.
30. Kelfkens G, de Gruijl FR, van der Leun JC. Carcinogenesis by short and long wave ultraviolet A; papillomas versus squamous cell carcinomas. In Biological Response to Utraviolet A radiation, F Urbach ed., Valdenmar Publishing Company 1992; pp.285-94.
31. Sterenborg H.J.C.M. and van der Leun JC. Tumorigenesis by long wavelenght UVA. In Biological Response to Utraviolet A radiation, F. Urbach ed., Valdenmar Publishing Company 1992; pp. 295-300.
32. van der Leun JC. Interactions of UVA and UVB in photodermatology: what was photoaugmentation? In Biological Response to Utraviolet A radiation, F Urbach ed., Valdenmar Publishing Company, 1992; pp. 309-16.
33. Setlow RB, Grist E, Thompson K, Woodhead AD: Wavelenghts effective in induction of malignant melanoma. *Proc Natl Acad Sci USA* 1993; 90: 6666-70.
34. Westerdahl J., Olsson H, Masbäck A, Ingvar C, Jonsson N. Is the use of sunscreens a risk factor for malignant melanoma ? Melanoma Res., 1995; 1995, 5: 59-65.

35 Westerdahl J, Olsson H, Masbäck A, Ingvar C, Jonsson N, Brandt L. Use of sunbeds or sunlamps and malignant melanoma in souththern Sweden. *Am J Epidemiol* 1994; 140: 691-9.
36. Fisher MS, Kripke ML. Systemic alteration induced in mice by ultraviolet light irradiation and its relation to ultraviolet carcinogenesis. *Proc Natl Acad Sci (USA)* 1977; 74: 1688-92.
37. Noonan FP, De Fabo EC, Kripke ML. Suppression of contact hypersensitivity by UV radiation and its relation to UV-iduced suppression of tumor immunity. *Photochem Photobiol* 1981; 34: 683-90.
38. Kripke ML, Morison WL, Parrish JA. Systemic suppression of contact hypersensitivity in mice by psoralen plus UVA radiation (PUVA). *J Invest Dermatol* 1983; 81: 87-92.
39. Kripke ML. Immunological responsiveness induced by ultraviolet radiation. *Immunol Rev* 1984; 80: 87-102.
40. Aubin F, Kripke ML. Effects of ultraviolet A radiation on cutaneous immune cells. In Biological Response to Utraviolet A radiation, F Urbach ed., Valdenmar Publishing Company 1992; pp. 239-47.
41. Mutzhas MF, von Armin V, Hentschel HD, Volger E, Stickl HA. Effects of UVA 1 light on immune status in man. In Biological Response to Utraviolet A radiation, F Urbach ed., Valdenmar Publishing Company 1992; pp. 249-56.
42. Strauss GH, Greaves M, Price M, Bridges BA, Hall-Smith P, Vella-Biffa M. Inhibition of delayed hypersensitivity reaction in skin (DNCB test) by 8 methoxypsoralen photochemotherapy. *Lancet* 1980; 2: 556-9.
43. Moss C, Friedmann PS, Shuster S. Impaired contact hypersensitivity in untreated psoriasis and effects of photochemotherapy and dithranol/UVB. *Brit J Dermatol* 1981; 105: 503-508.
44. Aberer W, Schuler G, Stingl G, Hönisgmann H, Wolff K. Ultraviolet light depletes surface markers on Langerhans cells. *J Invest Dermatol* 1981; 76: 781-794, .
45. Koulu L, Christer T, Jansen CT, Viander M. Effect of UVA and UVB irradiation on human Langerhans cell membrane markers defined by ATPase activity and monoclonal antibodies (OKT 6 and anti-la). *Photodermatol* 1985; 2: 339-46.
46. Koulu L, Soderstrom KO, Jansen CT. Relation of antipsoriatic and Langerhans cell depleting effects of systemic psoralen photochemotherapy: a clinical, enzyme ,histochemical, and electron microscopic study. *J Invest dermatol* 1984; 82: 591-3.
47. Ashwoth J, Kahan MC, Breathnach L. PUVA therapy decreases HLA-DR, CD1a+ Langerhans cells and epidermal cell antigen-presenting capacity in human skin, but flow cytometrically-sorted residual HLA-Dr + CD1a+ Langehans cells exhibit normal alloantigen presenting function. *Br J Dermatol* 1989; 120:329-39.
48. Schartz W, Schell H, Huttnger G, Wasmeier H, Diepgen T. Effects of UVA on human stratum corneum histidine and urocanic acid isomers. *Photodermatol* 1987; 4: 269-71.
49. Harriot-Smith TG, Halliday WJ. Suppression of contact hypersensitivity by short term ultraviolet irradiation. II. The role of urocanic acid. *Clin Exp Immunol* 1988; 72: 174-7.
50. Elmets C.A., Bergstresser PR, Tigelaar RE, Wood PJ, Streilein JW. Analysis of the mechanism of unresponsiveness produced by haptens painted on skin exposed to low dose ultraviolet radiation. *J Exp Med* 1983; 158: 781-794.
51. Schwarz T. Mechanisms of UV-induced immunosuppression: Link between UV-induced tolerance and apoptosis. *Eur J Dermatol* 1988; 8: 196-197.
52. Schwarz A, Grabbe S, Rieman H, Aragane Y, Simon M, Manon S, Andrade S, Luger T, Zlotnik A, Schwarz T. In vivo effects of interleukin-10 on contact hypersensitivity and delayed-type hypersensitivity reactions. *J Invest Dermatol* 1994; 103, 211.
53. Scholzen T, Armstrong C, Luger T, Ansel JC. Neuropeptides in the skin: interactions between the neuroendocrine and the skin immune system. *Exp Dermatol* 1998; 7, in press.
54. Applegate L.A., Ley R.A., Alcaday J. and Kripke M.L.: Identification of the molecular target for the suppression of contact hypersensitivity by ultraviolet radiation. *J Exp Med* 1989; 170: 1117.
55. Kripke ML, Cox PA, Alas LG, Yarosh DB. Pyrimidine dimers in DNA initiate systemic immunosuppression in UV-irradiated mice. *Proc Natl Acad Sci USA* 1992; 89: 7516.
56. Krutmann J. Ultraviolet A radiation-induced immunomodulation: molecular and photobiological mechanisms. *Eur J Dermatol* 1998; 8: 200-2.
57. Meunier L. Photoprotection and photoimmunosuppression in man. *Eur. J. Dermatol* 1998; 8: 207-8.

58. Moyal D. Immunosuppression induced by chronic ultraviolet irradiation in humans and its prevention by sunscreens. *Eur J Dermatol* 1998; 8: 209-11.
59. Gould JW, Mercurio MG, Elmets CA. Cutaneous photosensitivity diseases induced by exogenous agents. *J Am Acad Dermatol* 1995; 33: 551-76.
60. Harber LC, Baer RL. Pathogenic mechanisms of drug-induced photosensitivity. *J Invest Dermatol* 1972; 58: 327-42.
61. Duteil L, Queille-Roussel C, Richard A, Rougier A, Ortonne JP: High protective effect of UVA filter reinforced sunscreens against phototoxicity of chlorpromazine and benzoyl peroxyde. *Am Acad Dermatol* 1998; Orlando.
62. Pao C, Norris PG, Corbett M, Hawk JLM. Polymorphic light eruption: prevalence in Australia and England. *Br J Dermatol* 1994; 130: 62-4.
63. Jeanmougin M, Civatte J. Benign summer light euption: a new entity? *Arch Dermatol* 1986; 122: 376.
64. D. Dubois D, Lacour JP, Ortonne JP. The melasma. In The european file of side effcts in dermatology 5th ed. A guide to drug eruption., W. Bruisma ed., BEDC 1985; 10: 23-8.
65. Lehmann P, Hölzle E, Kind P, Goerz G. Experimental reproduction of skin lesions in lupus erythematosus by UVA and UVB radiation. *J Am Acad Dermatol* 1990; 22: 181-7.
66. Moyal D, Cesarini JP, Binet O, Hourseau C. Reproduction "indoor" de la lucite estivale benigne. Mise en evidence de l'efficacité d'une crème possédant un fort pouvoir protecteur UVA. *Nouv Dermatol* 1992; 11: 349-52.
67. Callen JP, Roth DE, McGrath C, Dromgoole SH. Safety and efficacy of a broad-spectrum sunscreen in patients with discoid or subacute cutaneous lupus erythemtosus. *Cutis* 1991; 47: 130-6 .
68. Stege H, Ahrens A, Billmann-Eberwein C., Ruzicka T, Rougier A, Krutmann J. Pretreatment of human skin with a sunscreen or dihydroxy-acetone prevents photo-provocation-induced polymorphous light eruption and keratinocyte ICAM-1 expression. 19th World Congress of Dermatology 1997; Sydney.
69. Peyron JL, Raison-Peyron N, Meynadier J, Moyal D, Rougier A, Hourseau C. Prevention of solar urticaria using a broadspectrum sunscreen and determination of a solar urticaria protection factor (SUPF). 19th World Congress of Dermatology1997; Sydney.
70. Diffey BL, Stokes RP, Forestier S, Mazilier C, Rougier A. Suncare product photostability: a key parameter for a more realistic *in vitro* efficacy evaluation. *Eur J Dermatol* 1997; 7: 226-8.

Population exposure to solar UVA radiation

B.L. Diffey

B.L. Diffey: Medical Physics Department, General Hospital, Newcastle NE4 6BE, UK.

An essential factor in evaluating the consequences of UVA radiation on the skin is to consider the extent to which people are exposed. Whilst there are a number of artificial sources of UVA, most notably sunbeds for cosmetic tanning, by far the most common source is sunlight, and in this presentation I shall discuss the magnitude and variability of this exposure.

The solar ultraviolet radiation (UVR) to which an individual is exposed depends upon: (1) ambient UVR; (2) the fraction of UVR ambient received at different anatomical sites; (3) time spent outdoors. The UV dose absorbed by the skin is further modified by the use of photoprotective agents such as hats, clothing and sunscreens.

The daily ambient UVA measured by the author *(Fig. 1)* shows a summer to winter ratio of about 10:1, with day-to-day variations as a result of cloud cover. However, population UVA exposure will be subject to even greater variation owing to differences in individual behaviour. Estimates of personal exposure are best obtained by direct measurement using UV sensitive film badges

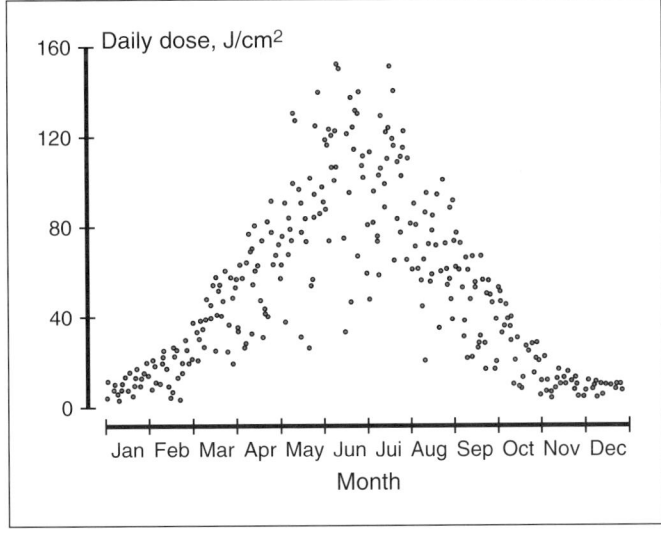

Figure 1. *Ambient UVA at Durham (55° N) during 1994.*

(see, for example [1-3]), or UV data loggers [4]. In general, these studies have been limited to monitoring the exposure of a few tens of people over periods ranging from a few hours to a few weeks. In order to determine the variability of exposure of different members of a population, direct measurement demands high compliance over an extended period of time by a large number of people. As yet, the largest personal dosimetry study reported the exposure of 180 children and adolescents over a 3-month period in different regions of England [5].

An alternative approach is to model the variables which affect personal exposure. In this approach, reported studies [6, 7] have taken a "typical" individual (*e.g.* outdoor worker) and estimated how long he spends outdoors in hourly intervals throughout the day for different months of the year. Whilst this method has been shown to give results in good agreement with the average obtained from personal dosimetry studies for similar exposure scenarios, it does not yield information about the variability in exposure of members of the same population, such as the "population" of British adult indoor workers. Furthermore, it is possible that taking an "average" person may be representative of nobody if the modes for a given measurement are grouped on either side of the mean [8].

The method adopted here has been to combine climatological data of UVA throughout the year (taking into account cloud cover) with the perceived behaviour of English adults who work indoors, to arrive at estimates of the variability of ultraviolet exposure of the face. One hundred and twenty adults (mean age 38 years; range 17-62 years; 68 male) were asked to imagine there are 100 people who work indoors in places such as factories, offices, shops and hospitals. Using their judgement they estimated how many of the 100 people spend less than 30 min outside on a typical weekday (Monday to Friday) in winter, how many spend between 30 min and 1 h outside, how many between 1 and 2 h, 2 and 4 h, 4 and 6 h, and more than 6 h. Outside in this context meant being in the open air; travelling in a car or being in a shop counted as being inside. Estimates were also made for a typical summer weekday (Monday to Friday), a typical winter weekend day (either a Saturday or a Sunday), a typical summer weekend day (Saturday or Sunday), and for 100 people who go on a summer holiday to somewhere sunny.

The average percentage of people who spend different time periods outdoors for each of these scenarios estimated by the 120 subjects is summarised in *Table I*.

By combining these average estimates with the day-to-day variability in ambient UVA, it is possible to calculate person-al UVA exposure for different periods of the year *(Fig. 2)*.

In *Figure 2* the data are described by box and whisker plots. The box represents the distance between the first and third quartiles with the median between them indicated by the horizontal line. The full range is encompassed between the top and bottom whiskers. In making the calculations, the exposure of the face is taken as 25% of ambient UVA; a fraction obtained from several studies of the anatomical distribution of sunlight. It is clear from *Figure 2* that there are large sea-

Table I. *Average estimated percentage of indoor workers who spend different time periods outdoors*

	< 0.5 h	0.5-1 h	1-2 h	2-4 h	4-6 h	> 6 h
Winter weekday	36	35	18	8	3	0
Summer weekday	11	18	27	25	13	6
Winter weekend	16	23	26	20	11	4
Summer weekend	4	8	17	24	27	20
Summer holiday	0	2	5	14	29	50

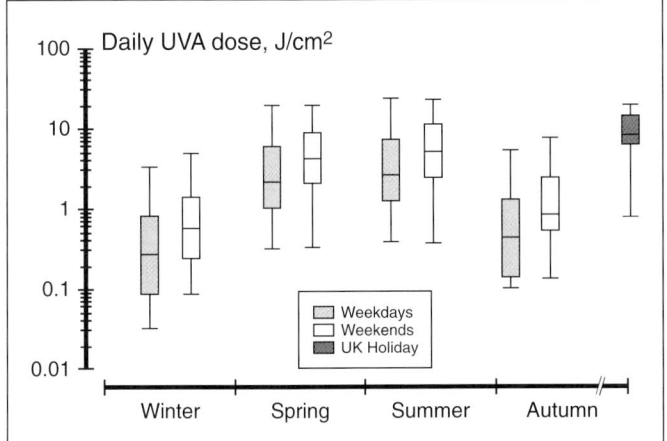

Figure 2. *Daily solar UVA dose in British indoor workers.*

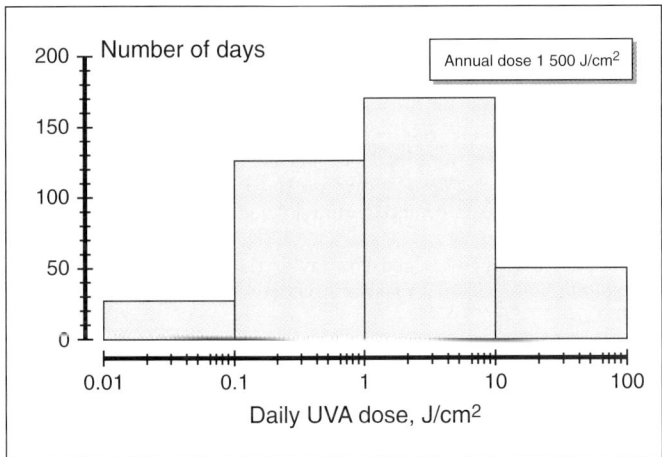

Figure 3. *Solar UVA dose in indoor workers including weekend and vacation exposure.*

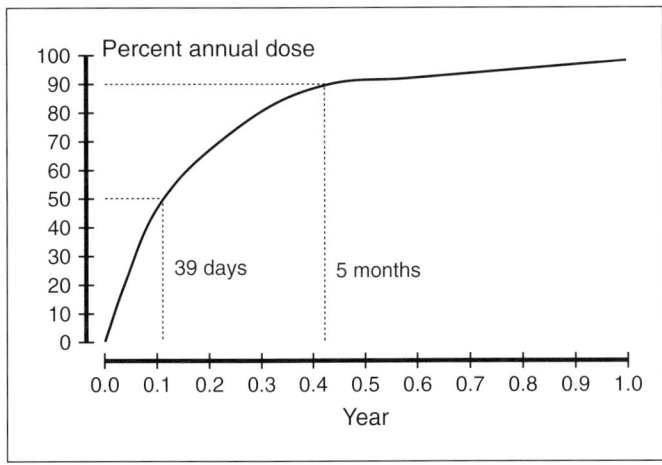

Figure 4. *Ranked daily solar UVA doses in indoor workers.*

sonal variations in personal UVA exposure which are due not only to seasonal changes in ambient UVA, but just as importantly to seasonal variation in behaviour (see *Table I*). Not surprisingly, holiday exposure accounts for the largest daily UV doses. Whilst there is only a 10-fold difference in clear sky, daily UVA from mid-winter to mid-summer, there is something like a 1,000-fold variation in the daily personal dose throughout the year *(Fig. 3)*, with a dose to the face of between 1 and 10 J/cm^2 on about half the days a year. If the daily personal UVA doses are ranked *(Fig. 4)*, we can see that 50% of annual personal exposure of approximately 1,500 J/cm^2 is received on just 39 days per year, and that the cumulative exposure for 7 months each year only contributes about 10% of our annual dose. In conclusion, this analysis questions the need for year-round UVA absorbers in day care products.

References

1. Challoner AVJ, Corless D, Davis A, Deane GHW, Diffey BL, Gupta SP, Magnus IA. Personnel monitoring of exposure to ultraviolet radiation. *Clin Exp Dermatol* 1976; 1: 175-9.
2. Slaper H. *Skin cancer and UV exposure: investigation of the estimation of risks*. PhD Thesis, University of Utrecht, The Netherlands, 1987.
3. Gies HP, Roy CR, Toomey S, Mac Lennan R, Watson M. Solar UVR exposures of three groups of outdoor workers on the Sunshine Coast, Queensland. *Photochem Photobiol* 1995; 62: 1015-21.
4. Diffey BL, Saunders PJ. Behaviour outdoors and its effect on personal ultraviolet exposure rate measured using a portable data logging dosimeter. *Photochem Photobiol* 1995; 61: 615-8.
5. Diffey BL, Gibson CJ, Haylock R, McKinlay AF. Outdoor ultraviolet exposure of children and adolescents. *Br J Dermatol* 1996 (in press).
6. Rosenthal FS, West SK, Munoz B, Emmett EA, Strickland PT, Taylor HR. Ocular and facial skin exposure to ultraviolet radiation in sunlight: a personal exposure model with application to a worker population. *Health Physics* 1991; 61: 77-86.
7. Diffey BL. Stratospheric ozone depletion and the risk of non-melanoma skin cancer in a British population. *Phys Med Biol* 1992; 37: 2267-79.
8. Martin P, Bateson P. *Measuring behaviour: an introductory guide*. Cambridge: Cambridge University Press, 2nd edition, 1993: 13-4.

Influences of UVA
in experimental photocarcinogenesis

P. Donald Forbes

P.D. Forbes: Director of Photobiology, Argus Research Laboratories, Inc., Genzyme Transgenics Corp., 905 Sheehy Drive, Horsham, PA 19044, USA.

A significant amount of new information is available on cutaneous effects of solar radiation, but we are left with many uncertainties about prevention or reversal of damage caused by "light" exposure. This is partly because of questions about the influence of that part of the solar spectrum from approximately the end of the visible portion (*i.e.*, wavelength 400 nm radiation) down to approximately 320 nm (*i.e.*, UVA).

Some of the concerns relate to two popular but inherently contradictory fashions: the acquisition and maintenance of a robust, active outdoor, tanned appearance, and the prevention or at least symptomatic reduction of the signs of chronic skin damage by solar radiation. These fashions both result from and influence the economics of clothing styles, of leisure travel and transportation, of resort, spa and health club operation, of cosmetic formulating, and of special lamp manufacturing.

Under some conditions and for some skin types, tanning and a variety of other cutaneous reactions can be induced by UVA alone, or in combination with UVB (< 320 > 280 nm). There are economic incentives in maximizing the "benefit" (tanning) part of this equation; there are health incentives in determining whether the tan imparts attributes other than cosmetic, and whether skin reactions that accompany the tanning process constitute significant risk. Businesses that promote tanning, travel and liesure activities often actively motivate people to increase their UVR exposures. For parts of the population, other sources of added ultraviolet radiation include indoor illumination (particularly from fluorescent and discharge lamps), industrial irradiation devices, and clinical phototherapy, photochemotherapy and photodynamic therapy.

It is probably useful to think of parts of the UV spectrum as components of a treatment mix, where each item has the potential for both useful and harmful effects. As toxicologists like to paraphrase, "the devil is in the dose", and at some dose, perhaps a greatly exaggerated one, almost anything can have toxic effects. With UVA, for example, it is not enough simply to demonstrate the possibility of a biological response; it is essential to determine whether a response of any relevance results from a plausible dose. So, what are the advances in understanding UVA effects in photocarcinogenesis, and where are our principal uncertainties? Here are examples.

The published literature now contains abundant data on experimental photocarcinogenesis, mainly in rodents. What do the data appear to tell us about UVB *versus* UVA effects?

First of all, the tumorigenic effects of solar radiation, when UVB is present, is strongly dominated by the UVB component; in the hairless mouse model, the UVA contribution to effectiveness (expressed as median time to tumor) is significant only when the UVB component represents less than 2% of the total UVR [1]. Secondly, UVA alone can produce skin tumors in mice, and the dose relationships are quite well defined [2, 3]. In reality, repeated exposures to skin rarely involve absolutely clean sources of UVA. When, in a mixed spectrum, the dose fraction represented by UVA is a substantial part of the total, then the effective radiation dose is additive across the UVA and UVB wavebands (*i.e.*, the effect caused by the UVA part will simply add to that caused by the UVB part) [4]. Neither a substantial protective nor synergistic influence by UVA has been convincingly demonstrated in experimental photocarcinogenesis. The idea of "photoaugmentation", was, to quote Van der Leun, "... at variance with careful observation and finally laid to rest in photobiology's graveyard of great misunderstandings" [5].

Thirdly, while some contribution of UVA tumorigenic effectiveness in a solar spectrum is generally accepted as a reality, the definition of a single, reliably quantitative weighting function has been elusive. This is due, in part, to different assumptions about the most appropriate endpoint. It is convenient to use median time to tumor in laboratory studies with mice. However, if rather than 50% prevalence, one chooses 5% or 1% (*i.e.*, more like the levels encountered in epidemiological studies), the slopes of dose response curves for UVB and 365 nm radiation are not parallel. This implies that the relative carcinogenicity of the two types of radiation depends on the level at which the comparison is made [2]. The most conservative working solution may be to settle on a smooth weighting function that decreases with increasing wavelength in the UVB and then flattens out, beginning at just above 335nm. This would provide, for each wavelength in the UVA-1 region (*i.e.*, 340-400 nm), an estimate of slightly less than 10^{-3} times the peak effectiveness found at about 295 nm.

Aging changes and tumorigenesis are at least temporally related. Are they separable in terms of induction mechanism, as cosmetic counter advertising would lead us to believe (*i.e.*, that UVB comprises the "sunburn rays", but UVA "causes aging")?

The Bissett model [6] attributes a significant portion of at least one "aging" endpoint in hairless mice to UVA, although this view is not supported by the hairless mouse study of Wulf *et al.* [7]. Bernstein's papers [8-10], based on models using the human elastin promoter gene *in vitro* and *in vivo*, show a very significant impact of solar radiation, with virtually all of the effect accounted for by the UVB component.

How does product photodegradation or photosensitization bear on the issues of photocarcinogenesis?

At the very least, photodegradation may mean loss of a primary substance such as UV absorber; secondary effects might include accelerated loss of other substances, or the appearance of chemically or biologically significant photoproducts. Loss of one or more absorbers implies loss of protection; the significance of this could be a function of the kinetics.

Photosensitization may be inadvertent or intentional; the safety consequences are quite different for porphyrins, phthalocyanines, psoralens and fluoroquinolone antibiotics. Sunscreens have been suggested as possibly extending the usefulness of photosensitizing drugs in a clinical setting, but relatively low protective factors in the UVA region would appear to limit this application.

Does UVA have a unique bearing on the role of photoimmunology in photocarcinogenesis?

Current evidence indicates: (1) that UV exposure of skin can influence aspects of both topical and systemic immune sensitization; and (2) that the immune system can influence the expression of photocarcinogenesis in mice. The most recent quantitative data argue that, across the UV spectrum, the effectiveness of wavebands in suppressing delayed contact sensitization is dominated by the wavelenghs that producted edema or erythema [11]. Again, this would appear to support the concept that a detectable UVA contribution to effectiveness would only be expected when exogenous photosensitization occurs, or when the dose fraction represented by UVA is a substantial part of the total (*e.g.*, with tanning bed exposure).

References

1. Cole CA, Forbes PD, Davis RE. An action spectrum for photocarcinogenesis. *Photochem Photobiol* 1986; 43: 275-84.
2. De Gruijl FR, Sterenborg HJCM, Forbes PD, Davies RE, Cole C, Kelfkens G, van Weelden H, Slaper H, van der Leun JC. Wavelength dependence of skin cancer induction by ultraviolet irradiation of albino hairless mice. *Cancer Research* 1993; 53: 53-60.
3. De Gruijl FR, Forbes PD. UV-induced skin cancer in a hairless mouse model. *BioEssays* 1995; 17: 651-60.
4. Forbes PD. Relative effectiveness of UVA and UVB for photocarcinogenesis. In: *The biological effects of UVA radiation.* Urbach F, Gange RW, eds. New York: Praeger Publishers, USA, 1986.
5. Van der Leun JC. Interactions of UVA and UVB in photodermatology: what was photoaugmentation? In: *Biological responses to ultraviolet A radiation.* Urbach F, ed. Kansas: Overland Park, Valdenmar Publishing Co, USA, 1992.
6. Bissett DL, Hillegrand GG, Hannon DP. The hairless mouse as a model of skin photoaging: its use to evaluate photoprotective materials. *Photodermatology* 1989; 6: 228-33.
7. Wulf HC, Poulsen T, Davies RE, Urbach F. Narrow-band UV radiation and induction of dermal elastosis and skin cancer. *Photodermatology* 1989; 6: 44-51.
8. Bernstein EF, Chen YQ, Tamai K, Shepley KJ, Resnik KS, Zhang H, Tuan R, Mauviel A, Uitto J. Enhanced elastin and fibrillin gene expression in chronically photodamaged skin. *J Invest Dermatol* 1994; 103: 182-6.
9. Bernstein EF, Fisher LW, Li K, Lebaron RG, Tan EML, Uitto J. Differential expression of the versican and decorin genes in photoaged and sun-protected skin. *Laboratory Investigation* 1995; 72: 662-9.
10. Bernstein EF, Brown DB, Urbach F, Forbes D, Monaco MD, Wu M, Katchman SD, Uitto J. Ultraviolet radiation activates the human elastin promoter in transgenic mice: a novel *in vivo* and *in vitro* model of cutaneous photoaging. *J Invest Dermatol* 1995; 105: 269-73.
11. Roberts LK, Beasley DG, Learn DB, Giddens LD, Beard J, Stanfield JW. Ultraviolet spectral energy differences affect the ability of sunscreen lotions to prevent ultraviolet radiation-induced immunosuppression. *Photoderm Photobiol* 1996 (in press).

Photocarcinogenesis by UVA (365-nm) radiation

Annemarie de Laat, Henk J. van Kranen, Jan C. van der Leun,
Frank R. de Gruijl

A. de Laat, H.J. van Kranen, J.C. van der Leun, F.R. de Gruijl: Dermatology, University Hospital AZU, Utrecht, The Netherlands.

The relationship between tumor induction time, daily dose and wavelength by been determined in hairless mice with broadband UVB/UVA sources. After eliminating benign papillomas from the data (prevalent with UVA-dominated sources) the median induction time for carcinomas (and precursors) is inversely proportional to the daily dose to the power r ≈ 0.6; the tumor multiplicity rises with time to the power p ≈ 7 (6-9). Here we report on a tumor induction experiment which was conducted in order to determine whether these relationships apply in the near UVA spectrum. In our study, we also investigated the frequency and type of UVA (365-nm)-induced *p53* mutations. We found a lower dose dependency for tumor induction with UVA I radiation (r ≈ 0.4) compared with UVB radiation. The p53 mutation frequency in UVA I-induced tumors (four times fewer than in UVB-induced tumors) also appeared to drop, going from UVB to UVA.

Much information exists on UVB carcinogenesis: on the relevant DNA damage, cellular responses, repair mechanisms, frequency and spectrum of *p53* mutations, and the dose-response relationship for tumor induction. Part of the human UV-induced skin cancer risk stems from longwave UVA exposure, both from natural and from artificial sources, but the relevance and mechanisms of UVA carcinogenesis are far less well understood than those of UVB carcinogenesis. Our aim was to acquire more information on tumor induction with longwave UVA radiation in terms of the relationship between dose and tumor induction times in order to be able to define the wavelength dependency for tumor induction with UV radiation more accurately. We also wanted some insight into the molecular pathways involved in UVA I carcinogenesis by studying *p53* mutations in UVA I- induced tumors. We therefore performed a tumor induction experiment with hairless mice, chronically irradiated with UVA I radiation from custom-made sources.

Materials and methods

Albino hairless mice (SKH:HR1) were irradiated daily with a custom-made, Philips 365-nm source (mercury arc, rigorously low- and high-cut filtered at 350 and 400 nm, respectively, isolating the 365-nm line). Four groups of 24 mice were irradiated daily for 2 h and received a daily dorsal dose of 75, 140, 240 and 430 kJ/m^2. The highest dose was 0.6 of the dose causing acute effects such as edema and erythema. One group of 16 mice served as an non-irradiated control, and another group of 16 mice was used as a positive control for UVB exposure and received a daily dorsal dose of 920 J/m^2 from North American Philips F40 sunlamps.

The prevalence curves are fitted with Weibull cumulative probability curves, which are characterized by the time to 63% tumor bearing prevalence, and a steepness parameter, p (corresponding to the power of the time with which the tumor multiplicity rises). Median induction times were determined from log-normal fits to the prevalence data.

Results and discussion

Dose-time relationship

The highest UVA I dose group had to be abandoned prematurely because of severe scratching 3 months later (no tumors). In the other dose groups scratching occurred later and less frequently. The interference with tumor development was less and the effect was further minimized by removing an animal from the experiment if the scarred area became too large. The prevalences for non-papillomas in the three UVA I-irradiated groups showed a time course that was very similar to that observed in the present UVB-irradiated control group *(Fig. 1)*. The steepness of these curves (presented by p) is thought to be related to the number of rate limiting steps in the carcinogenic process. The average steepnesses of these prevalence curves are not significantly different between UVA I ($p = 5.7 \pm 1.4$) and UVB exposure ($p = 7.9 \pm 1.4$). The tumor kinetics for non-papilloma tumor induction were not significantly different from those found earlier with broadband UVB and UVA II-dominated

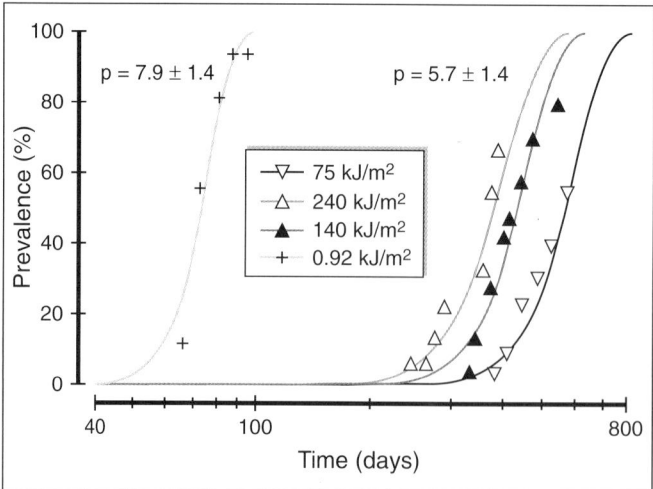

Figure 1. *Prevalences (percentages of tumor-bearing mice) for 1-mm non-papillomas versus time on a logarithmic scale in the daily UVB-exposed group (+ 0.92 kJ/m^2), and the daily UVA I-exposed groups (▲ 240 kJ/m^2, ▲ 140 kJ/m^2, ▲ 75 kJ/m^2). The drawn lines give the Weibull fits. The p represents the (average) steepness of the prevalence curve(s).*

sources, where p was in the range of 6 to 9, and therefore indicate no difference in the number of rate limiting steps between UVA and UVB carcinogenesis. The median tumor induction times (time point where 50% of the mice in a group are tumor bearing) varied from around 1 year in the 240-kJ/m^2 dose group to over 1 year and a half in the lowest 75-kJ/m^2 dose group. On the basis of these data we could determine a dose-time relationship for UVA carcinogenesis. The dose dependency of tumor induction with UVA I radiation appeared to be lower than with UVB radiation. The median induction time of carcinomas (and precursors) was inversely proportional to the daily UVA I exposure to the power $r \approx 0.4$, whereas with UVB and UVA II-dominated sources the r-value was 0.6. This difference implies that for carcinogenicity the ratio of UVA I over UVB will increase as the daily doses are lowered, and that this ratio cannot be presented by a single multiplicative factor in an action spectrum. *Figure 2* demonstrates this point by plotting the different relative carcinogenicities of three different daily UVA I (365-nm) exposures: the 365-nm carcinogenicity is found to be 0.6-0.9×10^{-4} times that at 293-nm, the wavelength of maximum carcinogenicity in hairless mice. This entire range is well within the margins of uncertainty of the earlier estimated

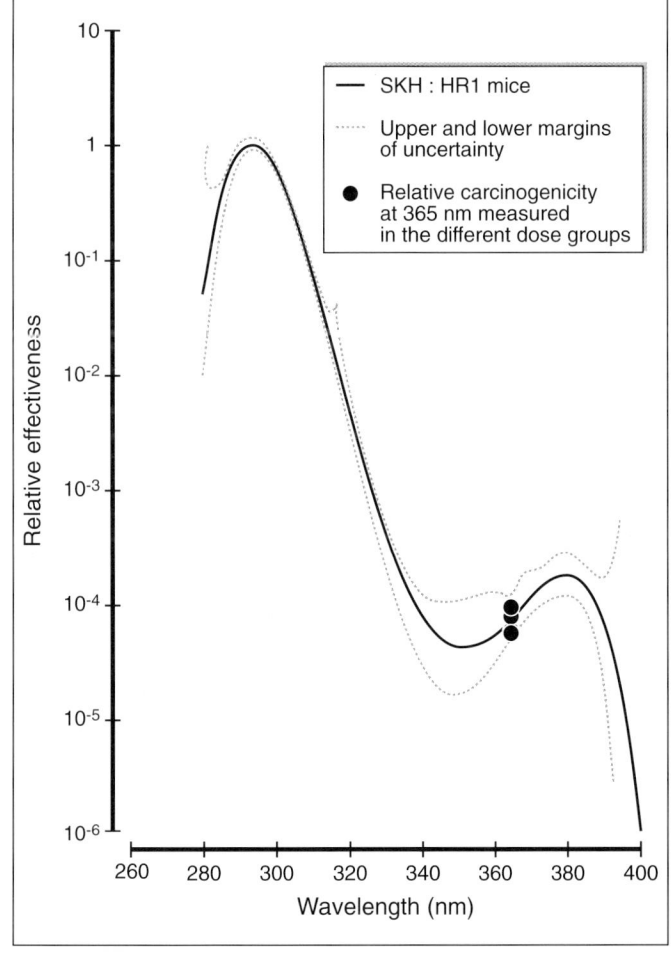

Figure 2. *Previously determined SCUP action spectrum for skin cancer induction in SKH:HR1 mice (—) with upper and lower margins of uncertainty (…) completed with present data on the relative carcinogenicities at 365 nm measured in the different dose groups (●). The relative carcinogenicity shifts from 0.56×10^{-4} in the 240-kJ/m^2 dose group to 0.77×10^{-4} in the 140-kJ/m^2 dose group up to 0.90×10^{-4} in the 75-kJ/m^2 dose group.*

SCUP$_m$ action spectrum in the UVA I region. Because of the deviating value of r, the previously determined additivity of carcinogenic UVA and carcinogenic UVB [1] becomes doubtful when the UV carcinogenicity is dominated by a UVA I contribution. Caution should therefore be exercised with an extrapolation of the carcinogenic risk in humans from UVB (sunlight) to that from UVA I (certain tanning lamps) exposure: the UVA exposure may well be more carcinogenic than anticipated.

According to the multistage theory, a lower dose dependency for UVA I could mean that the number of UV-driven steps is lower in UVA I carcinogenesis than in UVB carcinogenesis, *i.e.*, a step which is UV-driven in UVB carcinogenesis is not UV-driven in UVA I carcinogenesis. Either the step is absent in UVA I carcinogenesis or is driven by other UV-independent "background" processes, *e.g.*, oxidation from metabolic processes.

UVA I-induced *p53* mutations

To come to a meaningful extension of the action spectrum, the underlying differences between 365-nm and UVB in UV-driven processes need to be elucidated. Mutation spectra in oncogenes or tumor suppressor genes of skin tumors from mouse and man could provide basic information on this point. Unlike proto-oncogenes which require specific mutations to become activated, tumor suppressor genes can be inactived by a much broader range of mutations and thus retain more clearly the specific signature of the carcinogen. Signature mutations for UVB radiation, found both *in vitro* and *in vivo*, occur at dipyrimidine sites and they are C → T transitions and CC → TT tandem double mutations, most likely attributable to unrepaired cyclobutane pyrimidine dimers (CPD) and/or 6-4 photoproducts. The mutations induced by UVA I radiation are likely to be different from those induced by UVB because the initiating type of damage is likely to be different too. UVA I is known to act on DNA through interaction with "endogenous photosensitizers" that subsequently generate reactive oxygen species (ROS) [2]. Different types of damage have been reported after UVA irradiation (SSB - single strand breaks –, DPC – DNA protein crosslinks –, oxidative damages like adenine-oxide and 8 hydroxyguanine). Mutations corresponding to oxidative damage are expected after UVA I irradiation. In mammalian cells the T → G transversions are considered as UVA signature mutations [3]. We analyzed the conserved domains of the *p53* tumor suppressor gene in UVA I-induced tumors and found a much lower mutation frequency (6 out of 42) compared to that in UVB-induced tumors (54-73% mutated) [4], indicating that carcinogenic routes other than those involving *p53* mutations are more important with long-wave UVA carcinogenesis. UVA I-induced mutations were almost exclusively (6 out of 7) C → T transitions located at codon 267, the major UVB hotspot. No other mutations were found which could confirm previous results on other genes or which could be indicative of oxidative-induced damage as premutagenic lesions with UVA.

Conclusions

A larger number of UVA I-induced mutations are necessary to detect and characterize a possible involvement of ROS in UVA I carcinogenesis. It is hypothesized that under UVB exposure, *p53*-mutated cells have a developmental advantage over non-mutated cells and are more prone to further mutations. If UVA I is not capable of inducing these mutation, such a process will loose importance in UVA I carcinogenesis. Hence, the striking lack of *p53* mutations found in UVA I-induced tumors (four times fewer than in UVB-induced tumors) may well be related to the lower dose-dependency. The differences in types and processing of DNA damage induced by UVA or UVB exposure is likely to be at the core of the difference found in dose dependency of tumor induction.

Acknowledgements

We thank Anja de Vries and Joost Van der Ven for the *p53* mutation analyses. This work was partially supported by Philips Lighting and by the Environment Program of the European Community, Grant ENV4-CT96-0172.

References

1. Berg RJW, De Gruijl FR, Van der Leun JC. Interaction between ultraviolet-A and ultraviolet-B radiations in skin cancer induction in hairless mice. *Cancer Research* 1993; 53: 4212-7.
2. Tyrrell RM, Keyse SM. New trends in photobiology (invited review): the interaction of UVA radiation with cultured cells. *J Photochem Photobiol B* 1990; 4: 349-61.
3. Drobetsky EA, Turcotte J, Châteneauneuf A. A role for ultraviolet A in solar mutagenesis. *Proc Natl Acad Sci USA* 1995; 92: 2350-4.
4. Dumaz N, Van Kranen HJ, De Vries A, Berg RJW, Wester PW, Van Kreijl CF, Sarasin A, Daya-Grosjean L, De Gruijl FR. The role of UVB radiation in skin carcinogenesis through the analysis of *p53* gene mutations in squamous cell carcinomas of hairless mice. *Carcinogenesis* 1997 (in press).

Does UVA exposure cause human malignant melanoma?

Antony R. Young

A.R. Young: UMDS, Department of Dermatology, St Thomas' Hospital, London, UK.

Analysis of most human and mouse *in vivo* action spectrum studies for the harmful effects of UVR indicate that UVB is far more effective than UVA, usually by 2-4 orders of magnitude. Endpoints include, erythema, immunosuppression, non-melanoma skin cancer (NMSC) and photoageing. These results have been partially reassuring because, typically, less than 5% of solar UVR is UVB. Nonetheless, when such action spectra are used to generate biologically weighted effectiveness spectra it is clear that solar UVB causes about 80% of the effect in question. These studies and calculations have resulted in the general belief that protection from UVB, *e.g.* by sunscreens, would prevent most of the adverse effects of sunlight.

Conversely, they have tended to give rise to the belief that solar UVA poses no serious threat to human health. Some people have suggested that the greater skin penetration properties *per se* of UVA renders this part of the spectrum more likely to be the main cause of photoageing but this view, apart from being photobiologically naive, is not supported by action spectrum data.

Malignant melanoma – an important public health problem

The most serious effect of sunlight on human health is malignant melanoma (MM), the incidence of which has been increasing rapidly in most Western white-skinned populations over the past few decades. As with NMSC, sun-sensitive individuals who do not tan or tan poorly (types I and II respectively) are at greatest risk. Unlike NMSC, MM often occurs in young adults. As with NMSC, there is epidemiological evidence for a causal role of sunlight. Studies have shown that the pattern of solar exposure may be important. For recent reviews on MM in Scandinavia, Australia and North America, see Moan and Dahlback [1], Green and Williams [2] and Weinstock [3] respectively.

Which wavelengths cause malignant melanoma?

Epidemiology alone, no matter how solid the data, cannot identify solar wavelength dependence which may include visible radiation. Such information can come only from animal models. Studies in the marsupial *Monodelphis domestica* have indicated that repeated long-term exposure to broad spectrum UVB + UVA can induce MM [4]. To date, the only action spectrum study for melanoma has been in the fish model *Xiphophorus* [5]. These studies have shown that although UVB is more effective that UVA, the difference in efficacy is only about one order of magnitude. Consequently, if these data are used to generate biologically effective spectra and extrapolated to humans they indicate that solar UVA causes > 90% of MM. Such extrapolation, from fish to human, is very controversial and much more difficult to justify than say from mouse to human. However, the fish data raise the important hypothesis that solar UVA may be a major factor in human MM. There are no direct data to support this hypothesis, although it is possible to interpret some epidemiological data in this respect. For example, until relatively recently, European sunscreens were primarily chemical UVB filters. Their use, enabling prolonged solar exposure without UVB-induced sunburn, will have resulted in larger UVA exposure doses, even if sub-erythemal, than would otherwise be obtained. A recent case control study showed that sunscreen use was a risk factor for MM [6]. It is possible that this is because of greater UVA exposure. Sunbed or sunlamp use was also shown to be a risk factor for MM, especially in people younger than 30 years [7]. These users were more likely to have used modern sunbeds containing high levels of UVA radiation, although one cannot exclude a small and unknown UVB content.

What is the function of melanin?

The synthesis of melanin by melanocytes is induced by UVR, especially in skin types III and IV who tan well and are less prone to MM. However, melanogenesis is apparent histologically, even in skin types I without clinical evidence of a tan [8]. It is widely assumed that melanin is a photoprotective agent but there are relatively few experimental studies on the photobiological properties of melanin *in vivo*. Studies in human skin *in vivo* have shown that tanning, induced in skin types I and II by repeated exposure to solar simulated radiation (SSR), affords no protection from DNA photodamage by a subsequent challenge dose of SSR [8, 9]. A comparable protocol did result in photoprotection in skin types III and IV. Several studies have indicated that melanin may be a photosensitizing agent [10]. In this context, it is important to appreciate that the term melanin is misleading as it does not describe a single chemical entity but structurally different biomolecules whose photochemical and photobiological properties are poorly understood [11]. Eumelanins are insoluble black or brown pigments whereas pheomelanins are alkali soluble yellow to reddish brown pigments. Both types have been detected in human skin [12] with a trend for greater eumelanin content with increasing skin type (I → III) but pheomelanin content seemed to be independent of skin type. There is a general consensus that eumelanin is more photoprotective than pheomelanin, but this is not supported by a significant body of experimental data. It is also important to appreciate that the syntheses of different melanins are complex processes with many intermediates and metabolites which may undergo photochemical reactions. 5-S-cysteinyldopa (5-S-CD) is a major colourless metabolite which has been shown to be photochemically unstable in the presence of oxygen and UVA [13], although the biological significance of this in the skin is unknown. Recently it was reported that 5-dihydroxyindole-2-carboxylic acid (DICA), an intermediate in the biosynthesis of eumelanins, sensitizes single strand breaks in naked DNA with 313 nm (UVB) radiation, especially in the presence of oxygen [14]. 313 nm was chosen because it is the peak absorption of DICA but similar responses would be expected in the UVA region where it also absorbs.

Oxygen dependent UVA photosensitization reactions will cause qualitatively different types of DNA photodamage from that by direct UVB absorption by DNA, such as thymine dimers. In general, recent research focus, especially in skin *in vivo*, has been on UVB-type lesions and their consequences. Overall, the studies described above show that the photochemistry and photobiology of melanogenesis is complex with the potential to cause a wide range of effects, some of which may be relevant to the induction of MM. It has recently been suggested that the lack of MM in "black" albinos in Africa may be a consequence of amelanotic melanocytes [15].

Conclusion

It would be unwise to dismiss the possibility that UVA is a major cause of human malignant melanoma. A better understanding of the photochemical and photobiological properties of melanin, especially in human skin *in vivo*, is urgently required.

References

1. Moan J, Dahlback A. Ultraviolet radiation and skin cancer: epidemiological data from Scandinavia. In: *Environmental photobiology*. Young AR, Bj-orn LO, Moan J, Nultsch W, eds. New York: Plenum Press, 1993; 255-93.
2. Green A, Williams G. Ultraviolet radiation and skin cancer: epidemiological data from Australia. In: *Environmental photobiology*. Young AR, Bj-orn LO, Moan J, Nultsch W, eds. New York: Plenum Press, 1993; 233-54.
3. Weinstock M. Ultraviolet radiation and skin cancer: epidemiological data from the United States and Canada. In: *Environmental photobiology*. Young AR, Bj-orn LO, Moan J, Nultsch W, eds. New York: Plenum Press, 1993; 295-344.
4. Ley RD, Appelgate LA, Padilla R, Stuart TD. Ultraviolet radiation-induced malignant melanoma in Monodelphis domestica. *Photochem Photobiol* 1989; 50: 1-5.
5. Setlow RB, Grist E, Thompson K, Woodhead AD. Wavelengths effective in the induction of malignant melanoma. *Proc Nat Acad Sci USA* 1993; 90: 6666-70.
6. Westerdahl J, Olsson H, Måsbäck A, Ingvar C, Jonsson N. Is the use of sunscreens a risk factor for malignant melanoma? *Melanoma Res* 1995; 5: 59-65.
7. Westerdahl J, Olsson H, Måsbäck A, Ingvar C, Jonsson N, Brandt L, J-onsson P-E, Möller T. Use of sunbeds or sunlamps and malignant melanoma in Southern Sweden. *Am J Epidemiol* 1994; 140: 691-9.
8. Young AR, Potten CS, Chadwick CA, Murphy GM, Hawk JLM, Cohen AJ. Photoprotection and 5-MOP photochemoprotection from UVR-induced DNA damage in humans: the role of skin type. *J Invest Dermatol* 1991; 97: 942-8.
9. Potten CS, Chadwick CA, Cohen AJ, Nikaido O, Matsunaga T, Schipper NW, Young AR. DNA damage in UV-irradiated human skin *in vivo*: automated direct measurements by image analysis (thymine dimers) compared with indirect measurement (unscheduled DNA synthesis) and protection by 5-methoxypsoralen. *Int J Radiat Res* 1993; 63: 313-24.

10. Hill HZ. The function of melanin or six blind people examine an elephant. *BioEssays* 1992; 14: 49-56.
11. Prota G. Progress in the chemistry of melanins and related compounds. *Med Res Rev* 1988; 8: 525-56.
12. Thody AJ, Higgins EM, Wakamatsu K, Ito S, Burchill SA, Marks JA. Pheomelanin as well as eumelanin is present in human epidermis. *J Invest Dermatol* 1991; 97: 340-4.
13. Constantini C, D'Ischia M, Palumbo A, Prota G. Photochemistry of 5-S-cysteinyldopa. *Photochem Photobiol* 1994; 60: 33-7.
14. Routaboul C, Serepentini C-L, Msika P, Cesarini J-P, Paillous N. Photosensitization of supercoiled DNA damage by 5,6-dihydroxyindole-2-carboxylic acid, a precursor of eumelanin. *Photochem Photobiol* 1995; 62: 469-75.
15. Diffey BL, Healy E, Thody AJ, Rees JL. Melanin, melanocytes, and melanoma. *Lancet* 1995; 346: 1713.

UVA and oxidative stress

Louis Dubertret

L. Dubertret: Institut de Recherche sur la Peau, Hôpital Saint-Louis, 1, avenue Claude-Vellefaux, F-75475, Paris Cedex 10, France.

Various skin chromophores such as NADH or flavin are able to absorb UVA and cause oxidative stress leading to damage lipids, proteins and DNA. Experiments have been undertaken in order to better understand the oxidative stress induced by UVA:

(1) UVA can induce lipid peroxidation in cultured human fibroblasts in a dose-related fashion. Lipid peroxidation evaluated by the formation of thiobarbituric reactive substances is positively correlated to LDH release the supernatant which indicates cell membrane damage [1].

(2) Cell membranes of human fibroblasts are damaged by UVA irradiation as proved by the decrease of membrane fluidity. This damage is inhibited by vitamin E [2].

(3) UVA induces lipid peroxidation more efficiently in normal human fibroblasts than in human keratinocytes. This difference is not linked to the cellular content of total glutathione, superoxide dismutase, glutathione peroxidase or catalase [3].

(4) The action spectrum for UVA-induced lipid peroxidation in cultured human skin fibroblasts has been studied. UVB is more efficient than UVA regarding this damage. However, UVB is only 10 to 100 times more efficient than UVA for lipid peroxidation. This is in contrast with the usual ratio between the biological efficiency of UVA *versus* UVB which is usually 1/1,000 or 1/10,000. This indicates that, because of the greater amount of UVA at the earths surface, UVA is equally, or more effective in this respect than UVB under the normal conditions of sun exposure of humans [4].

(5) UVA strongly decreases the cellular content of catalase (up to 85%) and to a lesser degree of glutathione (up to 15%). Irradiated human fibroblasts, previously depleted of catalase by incubation with aminotriazole, do not exhibit an increased peroxidation. This indicates that catalase plays a minor role in the protection of human fibroblasts against UVA peroxidation [5].

(6) Studying SOD and catalase content of human fibroblasts from different normal cell lines and the efficiency of lipid peroxidation after UVA irradiation, we have shown that the extent of lipid peroxidation is correlated with the ratio of SOD to catalase. Thus, when this ratio increases, by increasing SOD or decreasing catalase before UVA irradiation, the peroxidation of lipids increases. This suggests the involvement of the superoxide anion with a decrease in the destruction of H_2O_2 produced after dismutation of the superoxide anion by the superoxide dismutase. This decrease in elimination of H_2O_2 by catalase increases the possibility of the occurrence of a Fenton reaction *via* the superoxide anion and H_2O_2 leading to the formation of the hydroxyl radical which is highly oxidasing [6].

(7) Low doses of UVA are able to decrease the processing of LDL and of epidermal growth factor by human fibroblasts and keratinocytes. The diacylglycerol formation induced by EGF is also inhibited. This effect is correlated with the appearance of lipid peroxidation products and is inhibited by vitamin E. This suggests a strong alteration *via* the oxidative stress induced by UVA, of the cell receptor-mediated endocytosis pathway [7, 8].

(8) With low doses of UVA irradiation, we observe a very early alteration of the actin structure using fluorescein-labelled phalloidin. This very early effect on the cytoskeleton could partly explain the alterations of the endocytotic processes [9].

(9) UVA inhibits diphosphatidylglycerol synthesis in NCTC 2,544 human keratinocytes. This participation of lipids specifically involved in mitochondrial membranes lead us to investigate the possible role of UVA on mitochondrial function [10].

(10) Lovastatin – an effective cholesterol synthesis inhibitor – enhances the cytotoxicity of UVA towards NCTC 2,544 human keratinocytes. This effect is prevented by cholesterol supplementation and by a cathepsin inhibitor. Lovastatin does not absorb light and is not toxic to these cell lines. This effect seems to be linked to a destabilization of the lysosomal membrane linked to a decrease in cholesterol synthesis. This increases the sensitivity of the lysosomal membrane to UVA. According to this indirect effect, it would be interesting to look at the effect of UVA on patients treated with lovastatin [11].

(11) Selenium is unable to protect normal human fibroblasts from damage by UVA, but human fibroblasts cultured in a medium depleted of selenium exhibit a strong increase in sensitivity. This increased sensitivity returns to normal after supplementation with selenium. Thus, the role of selenium and the control of the synthesis of stress proteins by selenium would be interesting to study [12].

(12) UVA efficiently inhibits antigen presentation by Langerhans cells in allogenic situations. This effect is correlated with the appearance of lipid peroxidation products and inhibited by pre-incubation with Vitamin E. This effect could be related to a decrease in the endocytotic functions of Langerhans cells perhaps mediated by the effect of UVA on the cytoskeleton [13].

(13) The effect of UVA and UVB on human cell-lines derived from 293 cells transfected with an Epstein-Barr virus-based shuttle vector harbouring the *lacZ'* bacterial gene as a mutagenic target has been studied. It is necessary to use an UVA dose 700 fold higher than UVB to induce identical alterations in cell survival. This UVA/UVB ratio is comparable to the one reaching the basal cell layer of the epidermis after sun exposure using a UVB sunscreen. The frequency of UVA- and UVB-induced mutations increased with UV dose. At cell survival higher than 10%, a similar frequency of mutations was found with UVA and UVB whereas for cell survival lower than 10%, UVA induced 2.3 more mutations than UVB. Mutations on the A/T are more frequently induced by UVA (41%) than by UVB (18%) [14].

In conclusion, UVA is very efficient at inducing oxidative stress in human fibroblasts and keratinocytes. This oxidative stress is responsible for the alterations of many cell functions leading to modifications of cell nutrition, of the sensitivity to growth factors and of the ability to present antigens. This oxidative stress is also able to induce mutations. This induction of mutations seems nearly as efficient as mutations induced by UVB under normal conditions of life on the earth surface.

However, many questions remain to be investigated: the effect of low irradiation rate *versus* high irradiation rate, the kinetics of induction of protective mechanisms *versus* the induction of cellular damage, the reversibility of UVA-induced cellular damage, the relative efficacy of different antioxidant mechanisms in the cells for preventing UVA attack, the effect of UVA on transduction signals, the identification of the endogenous chromophores responsible for the UVA peroxidation and, through all these studies, the ability to detect differences between individuals in order to detect persons at risks.

References

1. Morlière P, Moysan A, Santus R, Hüppe G, Mazière J-C, Dubertret L. UVA-induced lipid peroxidation in cultured human fibroblasts. *Biochim Biophys Acta* 1991; 1084: 261-8.
2. Gaboriau F, Morlière P, Marquis I, Moysan A, Gèze M, Dubertret L. Membrane damage induced in cultured human skin fibroblasts by UVA irradiation. *Photochem Photobiol* 1993; 98: 515-20.
3. Moysan A, Clément-Lacroix P, Michel L, Dubertret L, Morlière P. Effects of ultraviolet A and antioxidant defense in cultured fibroblasts and keratinocytes. *Photodermatol Photoimmunol Photomed* 1996 (in press).
4. Morlière P, Moysan A, Tirache I. Action spectrum for UV-induced lipid peroxidation in cultured human skin fibroblasts. *Free Radical Biology & Medicine* 1995; 19: 365-71.
5. Tirache I, Morlière P. Hydrogen peroxide and catalase in UVA-induced lipid peroxidation in cultured fibroblasts. *Redox Report* 1995; 1: 105-11.
6. Morlière P, Moysan A, Marquis I, Gaboriau F, Dubertret L. Peroxidation lipidique induite par les UVA et défenses antioxydantes induites chez les fibroblastes cutanés en culture. *Nouv Dermatol* 1994; 13: 317-8.
7. Djavaheri-Mergny M, Mazière C, Santus R, Dubertret L, Mazière J-C. Ultraviolet A decreases epidermal growth factor (EGF) processing in cultured human fibroblasts and keratinocytes: inhibition of EGF-induced diacylglycerol formation. *J Invest Dermatol* 1994; 102: 192-6.
8. Djavaheri-Mergny M, Mazière J-C, Santus R, Mora L, Mazière C, Auclair M, Dubertret L. Exposure to long wavelength ultraviolet radiation decreases processing of low density lipoprotein by cultured human fibroblasts. *Photochem Photomed* 1993; 57: 302-5.
9. Djavaheri-Mergny M, Pieraggi M-T, Mazière C, Santus R, Lageron A, Salvayre R, Dubertret L, Mazière J-C. Early alterations of actin in cultured human keratinocytes and fibroblasts exposed to long-wavelength radiations. Possible involvement in the UVA-induced perturbations of endocytic processes. *Photochem Photobiol* 1994; 59: 48-52.
10. Djavaheri-Mergny M, Mora L, Mazière C, Auclair M, Santus R, Dubertret L, Mazière J-C. Inhibition of diphosphatidylglycerol synthesis by UVA radiations in NCTC 2,544 human keratinocytes. *Biochem J* 1994; 599: 85-90.
11. Quiec D, Mazière C, Auclair M, Santus R, Gardette J, Redziniak G, Franchi F, Dubertret L, Mazière J-C. Lovastatin enhances the photocytotoxicity of UVA radiation towards cultured NCTC 2,544 human keratinocytes: prevention by cholesterol supplementation and by a cathepsin inhibitor. *Biochem J* 1995; 310: 305-9.
12. Moysan A, Morlière P, Marquis I, Richard A, Dubertret L. Effects of selenium on UVA-induced lipid peroxidation in cultured human fibroblasts. *Skin Pharmacol* 1995; 8: 139-48.
13. Clément-Lacroix P, Michel L, Moysan A, Morlière P, Dubertret L. UVA-induced immune suppression in human skin: protective effect of vitamin E in human epidermal cells *in vitro*. *Br J Dermatol* 1996; 134: 77-84.
14. Robert C, Muel B, Benoit A, Dubertret L, Sarasin A, Stary A. Cell survival and mutagenesis induced by ultraviolet A and ultraviolet B rays in a human cell line. *J Invest Dermatol* (in press).

In vivo biological effects of UVA and sunscreen efficacy studies

Anny M-A. Fourtanier

A.M.-A. Fourtanier: Life Sciences-L'Oréal Research, Centre Charles Zviak, 90, rue du Général Roguet, F-92583 Clichy Cedex, France.

During the past few years a new publication on the biological effects of UVA has appeared in the literature almost monthly. This clearly demonstrates a considerable amount of research activity on this topic.

The first studies on the effects of UVA were started in our research department as early as 1994, simultaneously with the development of new UVA filters. The first priority was the definition and development of suitable UVA sources and testing protocols. This was followed by long-term studies, such as photoaging [1], as well as short-term studies on erythema and pigmentation [2, 3].

Later, the emphasis switched to the assessment of cellular and molecular events such as DNA damage [4] and oxidative stress [5], in recent years attention had focused on studies on immunosuppression and skin cancer [6].

The first UVA sources were flluorescent tubes but these had the problem of low output and contamination by UVB. Xenon arc sources, with suitable filtration, were available but until about 2 years ago the exposure fields were very small and of uneven intensity. Xenon arc sources have considerable infrared output which has to be filtered. However, this decreases overall output and modifies the UVA spectrum. Metal halide lamps, initially designed to provide a UVA-I source, are now available with the full UVA spectrum although some spectral modifications are still desirable. These lamps are expensive but have the great advantage of a high output with a large exposure field. With a suitable source, the next consideration is the exposure protocols, such as dose, frequency and duration of exposure. One should keep in mind that experimental conditions should simulate the "in life" exposure, for example a summer time daily exposure of two minimal erythemal dose (MED) corresponds to 20 J/cm^2 of UVA, which is equivalent to one UVA MED for a skin type II person.

One of our interests has been to compare the photobiological effects of the complete solar UVR spectrum (290-400 nm) using solar simulated radiation (SSR) with the full UVA spectrum (320-400 nm). Our data show that the colour and kinetics of SSR and UVA-induced erythema and pigmentation are different. An immediate erythema with a brownish-red colour, is evident with UVA, whereas the SSR induced erythema appears 8 to 16 h after exposure and is a red colour. UVA-induces immediate pigment darkening (IPD) which persists for up to 7 days. This has a blue-grey colour in comparison with the yellowish-brown colour of a tan induced 48 to 72 h after SSR exposure. This phenomenon has been termed persistent pigment darkening and is now proposed for the assessment of UVA sunscreen protection factors [2, 3].

In the mouse, UVA induces about 25% of the number of pyrimidine dimers per equivalent edematous dose of SSR [4]. Furthermore, it alters the number and the morphology of Langerhans cells and induces apoptotic cells (sunburn cells), but to a lesser extent than SSR for an equivalent erythematous/edematous dose.

For an equivalent edema dose in mouse, SSR is more immunosuppressive (systemic contact hypersensitivity to dinitrochlorobenzene) than filtered FS 40 tubes; it can be supposed that UVA enhances the UVB effects.

UVA readily induces oxidative stress and hydroperoxides are found in the upper epidermis after low UVA dose. Catalase and ICAM-1 expression are depressed by UVA exposure [5].

It is thought that the acute effects of UVA contribute to the photoaging process in which changes such as skin sagging and loss of elasticity are observed [6, 7]. It is noteworthy that the chronic effects of UVA are barely distinguishable from those of SSR.

Our data show that sunscreens should offer good UVA protection. UVA filters such as Oxybenzone and Parsol® 1789 do not afford complete protection across the UVA spectrum but this can be improved with micronised pigments such as titanium dioxide. We believe that it is important to ensure that sunscreens offer the same level of protection across the 290-370 nm range. With this in mind, we have developed a new broad spectrum UVA filter called Mexoryl® SX which we have shown to be very effective in inhibiting a wide range of UVA-induced effects [6-9], as well as the effects of SSR. For example we have shown that it is more effective at preventing photocarcinogenesis by SSR than a UVB sunscreen, Octyl Methoxycinnamate [10]. Mexoryl® SX also performed better in SSR studies on the inhibition of pyrimidine dimers [4], Langerhans cell depletion, suppression of contact hypersensitivity and the photo-isomerization of urocanic acid [11].

Overall, although we have made considerable progress in our understanding of the effects of UVA and their prevention we still have a long way to go.

References

1. Boyer B, Fourtanier A, Kern P, Labat-Robert J. UVA and UVB induced changes in collagen and fibronectin biosynthesis in the skin of hairless mice. *J Photochem Photobiol B Biology* 1992; 14: 247-59.
2. Chardon A, Cretois I, Hourseau C. Skin colour typology and suntanning pathways or comparative colorimetric follow up on humans of the tanning induced by cumulative exposures to UVB, UVA and UVB + A radiations. *16th AFSCC Congress*; New York, Oct 8-10, 1990.
3. Chardon A, Moyal D, Hourseau C. Skin immediate pigment darkening applied to UVA protection assessment. *Photochem Photobiol* 1991; 53S: 115.
4. Ley R, Fourtanier A. Sunscreen protection against ultraviolet radiation (UVR)-induced pyrimidine dimers in mouse epidermal DNA. *Photochem Photobiol* 1996 (in press).
5. Treina G, Scaletta C, Fourtanier A, Seite S, Frenk E, Applegate LA. Expression of intercellular adhesion molecule-1 (ICAM) in UVA irradiated human skin cells in vivo. *Br J Dermatol* 1996 (in press).

6. Fourtanier A, Labat-Robert J, Kern P, Berrebi C, Gracia AM, Boyer B. In vivo evaluation of photoprotection against UVA irradiation by a new sunscreen Mexoryl® SX. *Photochem Photobiol* 1992; 55 (4): 549-60.
7. Fourtanier A, Labat-Robert J, Kern P. Effects of chronic suberythemal doses of pure UVA radiation-protective effect of a new sunscreen Mexoryl® SX. In: *Biological responses to ultraviolet A radiation*, Urbach F, ed. Overland Park: Valdenmar Publishing Company, 1992; 393-407.
8. Fourtanier A, Moyal D. la photoprotection apportée par un nouveau filtre UVA: le Mexoryl® SX. *L'Eurobiologiste* 1994; 28 (210): 25-31.
9. Moyal D, Seite S, Richard S, de Rigal J, Lévêque JL, Hourseau C, Fourtanier A. *Effect of repeated suberythemal doses of UVA in human skin and protection by Mexoryl® SX*. ESP Cambridge: UK, 1995.
10. Fourtanier A. Mexoryl® SX protects against solar simulated UVR induced photocarcinogenesis in mice. *Photochem Photobiol* 1996 (in press).
11. Krien PM, Moyal D. Sunscreen with broad-spectrum absorption decreases the trans to cis photoisomerization of urocanic acid in the human stratum corneum after multiple UV light exposures. *Photochem Photobiol* 1994; 60 (3): 280-7.

Molecular aspects of photoaging

Jouni Uitto, Douglas B. Brown, Francis P. Gasparro, Eric F. Bernstein

J. Uitto, D.B. Brown, F.P. Gasparro, E.F. Bernstein: Departments of Dermatology and Cutaneous Biology, and Biochemistry and Molecular Pharmacology, Jefferson Medical College, and the Jefferson Institute of Molecular Medicine, Thomas Jefferson University, 233 South 10th Street, Suite 450, Philadelphia, Pennsylvania, 19107, USA.

Evidence from several lines of investigation has indicated that extrinsic aging, when superimposed on the intrinsic aging processes, plays the major role in age-associated degenerative changes of the skin. The extrinsic aging is primarily due to ultraviolet irradiation (UV), and thus is known as photoaging. Histopathologic, immunohistochemical and ultrastructural observations have demonstrated that dermal accumulation of elastotic material is a characteristic feature of photoaging. Subsequent biochemical and molecular studies have revealed that activation of elastin gene expression, with enhancement of transcriptional activity of other extracellular matrix genes, is an early event in photoaging. Based on this premise, we have recently developed a line of transgenic mice, which expresses the human elastin promoter, linked to a chloramphenicol acetyltransferase reporter gene, in a tissue-specific and developmentally regulated manner. Exposure of the skin of these animals to UV, particularly UVB, resulted in enhancement of elastin promoter activation. Irradiation of fibroblast cultures established from the skin of these animals revealed a significant effect by UVB while UVA had no effect. However, exposure of the cultures to UVA together with 8-methoxypsoralen resulted in a marked enhancement of the activity. Collectively, our results confirm the role of UVB in the development of solar elastosis and further identify UVA as a contributing factor in vivo. The transgenic mouse model serves as a useful system to study mechanisms of cutaneous photoaging and provides a convenient model to test compounds that may protect the skin against photodamage.

Cutaneous aging consists of distinct processes due to either intrinsic or extrinsic factors [1]. The intrinsic aging processes, also known as innate or chronologic aging, probably affect the skin in a manner similar to the way they affect various internal organs. Several mechanisms have been advanced to explain the biological basis of innate aging, and some of them would also be applicable to the skin [2]. One of the postulated mechasnisms, the rate of living theory, is based on the Hayflick cell phenomenon, an observation that diploid cells (skin fibroblasts) in culture have a defined lifespan. Extension of this observation to the tissue level, together with depletion of the stem cell population in the skin, could explain the loss of proliferative capacity of cells and degenerative cutaneous changes. Another theory revolves around post-translational modification of structural proteins [3]. This suggestion is based on clinical observations in patients with poorly controlled diabetes mellitus. These patients, due to persistent hyperglycemia, depict non-enzymatic glucosylation of various extracellular proteins, including lens proteins and collagens, with development of premature aging manifestations, including lens cataracts and early atherosclerosis. Finally, age-associated differentiation of the cells with differential gene expression could contribute to the degenerative changes in the skin [4]. For example, the rate of collagen biosynthesis and elastin gene expression, as determined at the protein and messenger RNA levels, have been shown to decline with advancing age, providing an explanation for dermal atrophy and loss of elastic fibers in the protected areas of skin.

Extrinsic aging, *i.e.*, changes due to exposure to the environment, primarily to ultraviolet irradiation (UV), is superimposed on the innate aging of the exposed areas of skin. The extrinsic aging, also known as photoaging, is clinically, biologically, and molecularly distinct from innate aging [1]. For example, the age-associated cutaneous changes due to innate aging manifest clinically with fine wrinkling, apparent atrophy of dermis and loss of subcutaneous adipose tissue. In photodamaged skin, the wrinkles are coarse with distinct furrowing, and the skin appears thickened due to accumulation of elastotic material, clinically termed as solar elastosis. Thus, photoaging is clearly distinct from innate aging, and a general notion is that more that 80% of visible aging in the sun-exposed areas of skin, such as face, is due to photoaging.

Molecular basis of photoaging

The predominant histopathologic change in solar elastosis is an accumulation of elastotic material in the upper and mid reticular dermis [5] *(Fig. 1)*. This material has been called "elastotic" due to the fact that it stains positively with elastic stains, such as Verhoeff-van Gieson stain, and early biochemical studies demonstrated that elastin is a major component in solar elastosis [5]. However, subsequent inmunofluorescence studies have demonstrated that the elastotic material also contains elastin-associated microfibrils, as well as fibrillin, fibronectin, and various proteoglycan/glycosaminoglycan macromolecules, such as decorin and versican [6-10]. Since all these macromolecules are synthesized by cultured fibroblasts, it is conceivable that activation of the biosynthetic machinery of resident dermal fibroblasts results in accumulation of these components. It should be emphasized, however, that ultrastructural examination of the elastotic material fails to reveal the presence of normal elastic fibers with characteristic morphology. Instead, haphazardly organized elastic structures with a granular appearance are detected, with the absence of normal elastic fibers [5]. Thus, the elastotic material accumulating in solar elastosis is not functional in providing elasticity and resilience to the skin.

Elucidation of the molecular biology of elastin has provided the tools to probe elastin gene expression in cutaneous aging [11, 12]. For example, Northern hybridization of RNA isolated from fibroblast cultures established from sun-protected and sun-damaged skin or directly from the corresponding areas of the skin, has revealed that elastin mRNA levels are enhanced up to 5.3-fold, apparently reflecting enhanced transcription of the elastin gene [13] *(Fig. 2)*. Furthermore, transient transfections of cultured fibroblasts with human elastin promoter linked to a reporter gene (chloramphenicol acetyl transferase, CAT) have confirmed enhanced promoter activity in fibroblasts from the photodamaged area of skin *(Fig. 3)*.Thus, activation of elastin promoter can serve as a marker for events leading to accumulation of elastotic material in photodamaged skin.

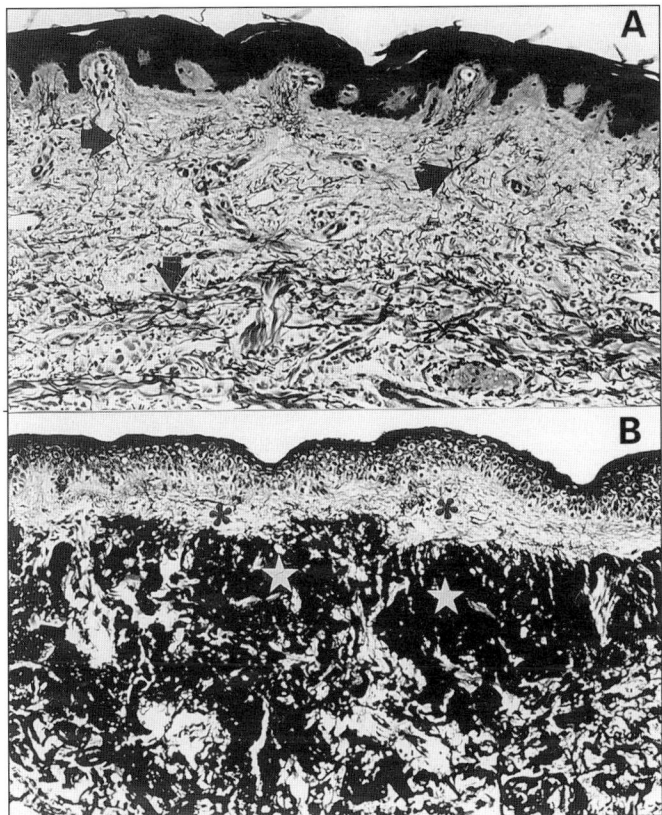

Figure 1. Demonstration of accumulation of the elastotic material in photodamaged skin. **(A)** In the dermis of the sun-protected area of skin (buttock), elastic fibers appear as thin structures (arrows), which are a minor components intertwined between collagen fibers. **(B)** In a sun-damaged area of the skin from the same individual (neck), mid-reticular dermis demonstrates massive accumulation of elastotic material (stars) which stains positively with Verhoeff-van Gieson stain. Note the "grenz-zone", devoid of elastotic material just below the epidermis in the upper papillary dermis (asterisks).

A novel transgenic mouse line as a model for photoaging

Previously, a variety of animal models have been used to study photoaging. Most of these models consist of irradiation of hairless mice or guinea pigs for extended periods with UV irradiation, and accumulation of elastin as determined by histochemical or immunohistological means to monitor the development of photoaging in the skin of these animals [14-18]. A distinct drawback of this model is that significant accumulation of elastin as a result of UV irradiation, depending on the wavelength, takes a relatively long time, and results from any pharmacological intervention studies are not immediately available.

As indicated above, our molecular studies have indicated that elastin promoter activity is markedly enhanced in photodamaged skin, and could consequently serve as a marker of activation of the processes leading to solar elastosis. On the basis of this premise, we have recently developed a transgenic mouse model for the assessment of mechanisms of photodamage [19]. Specifically, this homozygous transgenic mouse line has incorporated into its genome, 5.2 kb of the human elastin promoter linked to the CAT reporter gene [20]. CAT is a prokaryotic enzyme, not expressed in vertebrate animals, and consequently, assay of the CAT activity in the tissues of these mice directly reflects the activity of the human elastin promoter in the

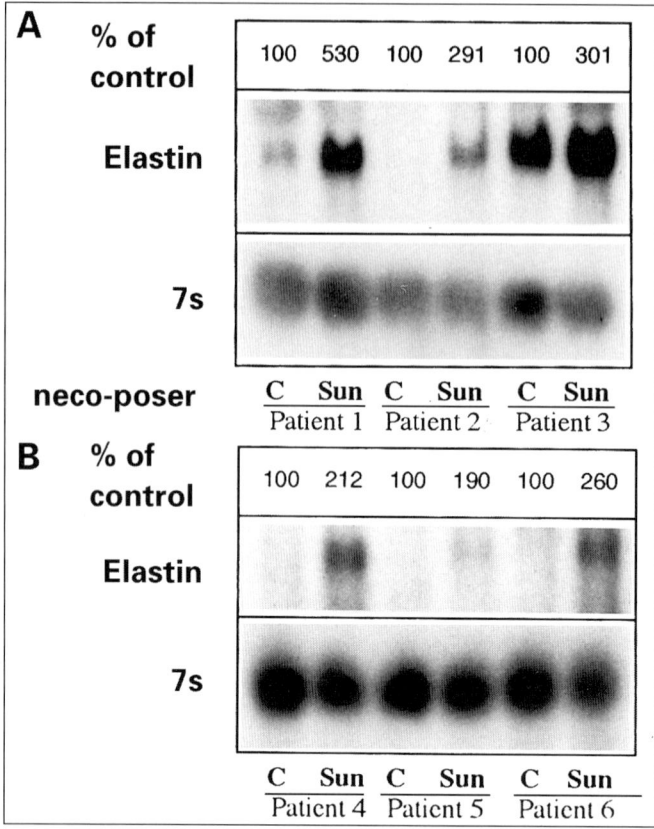

Figure 2. Demonstration of increased elastin mRNA levels in photodamaged skin. (A) Northern analysis, performed on pairs of first-passage fibroblast cultures established from three subjects, taken from photoaged neck skin (sun) or sun-protected buttock skin (C) of each subject, reveals a mean increase in elastin mRNA of 420% in photodamaged skin ($P < 0.01$). (B) Direct extraction of RNA from the tissue revealed a mean increase of 220% in elastin mRNA content as compared with sun-protected buttock skin ($P < 0.01$). All mRNA values are corrected for 7S ribosomal RNA content as shown on the lower panels (adapted from [13]).

mouse genome. During the validation process of this mouse model, it was noted that the human elastin promoter was expressed in a tissue-specific manner and the highest levels of expression were noted in the lungs and aorta, i.e., tissues endogenously active in elastin gene expression [20]. Furthermore, the promoter activity was developmentally regulated, the highest level of expression being noted during fetal and early postnatal periods with marked decline with the chronologic aging of the animals. These features suggested that the human elastin promoter present in the transgene behaves in a manner similar to the endogenous mouse elastin promoter [20]. We proposed, therefore, that this transgenic mouse model could serve as a model for studying mechanisms of photodamage to the skin [19].

Effects of UV irradiation on human elastin promoter activity

The validity of this transgenic mouse as a model of photoaging was initially tested by subjecting 4- or 5-day-old pups (before substantial hair growth) to UV-irradiation using UVA or UVB. For UVB, an array of seven Westinghouse FS40 sun lamps at the distance of 38 cm were used. As a source of UVA, seven Sylvania FR40T12 PUVA lamps in a similar array, filtered through window glass, was used. Irradiation of the mice *in vivo* with UVB demonstrated

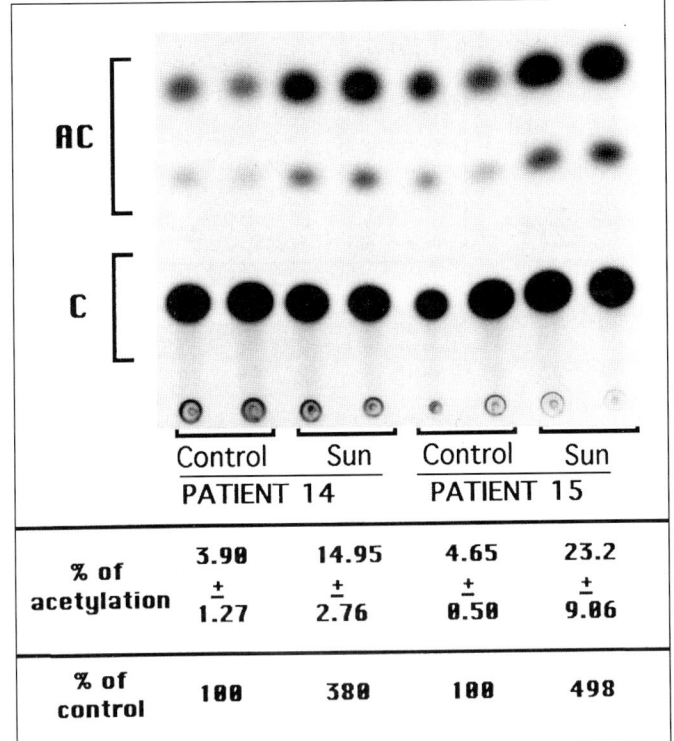

Figure 3. Demonstration of increased elastin promoter activity in first-passage cell cultures subjected to paired transient transfections with a human elastin promoter/CAT construct taken from photodamaged skin (sun), compared with cells from sun-protected sites in the same individuals (control). The increase in elastin promoter activity of 439% (P < 0.01) agrees well with the 420% increase in elastin mRNA levels demonstrated in parallel cultures from photodamaged skin, as shown in Figure 2 (adapted from [13]).

dose-dependent enhancement in elastin promoter activity [19]. A single dose of UVB (122.8 mJ/cm^2) resulted in 4.1-fold increase in relative activity of the promoter, and the 491.4 mJ/cm^2 resulted in 8.5-fold enhancement of the CAT activity *(Fig. 4A)*. Parallel irradiation with UVA resulted in a more modest, up to 1.8-fold increase with 38.2 J/cm^2 of UVA *(Fig. 4C)*. However, this small increase was reproducibly noted in several experiments [19].

To address the mechanisms of the elastin promoter activation by UVA *versus* UVB, fibroblast cultures established from the skin of the transgenic mice were similarly subjected to UV irradiation [19]. These *in vitro* studies revealed over 30-fold increases in the elastin promoter activity in response to UVB (5.5 mJ/cm^2), whereas no significant change in CAT activity was observed in response to UVA (2.2 J/cm^2) *(Fig. 4, B and D)*. These results suggested that UVB, which upregulated the elastin promoter both *in vivo* and *in vitro*, may have direct effects on dermal fibroblasts. On the other hand, UVA upregulated the elastin promoter at the fluences tested only *in vivo* but not *in vitro*, suggesting that the target for UVA irradiation *in vivo* is a cell other than the dermal fibroblast. A candidate cell is the epidermal keratinocyte which has been previously shown to release a variety of cytokines capable of enhancing elastin promoter activity *in vivo* using this transgenic animal model [21-23].

Since UVA clearly had an effect on human elastin promoter activity *in vivo*, although such activity was less dramatic than noted with UVB, we tested whether enhancement of UVA activity by 8-methoxypsoralen (8-MOP) in combination with UVA (PUVA) would be more

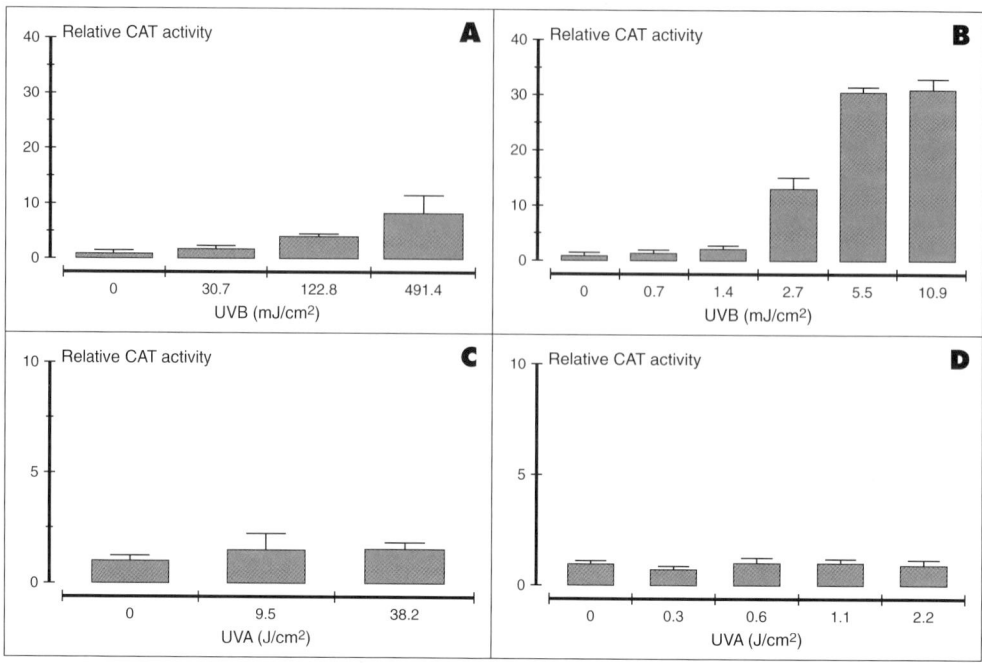

Figure 4. Effects of UVB and UVA on human elastin promoter activity in cultured fibroblasts from the skin of transgenic mice expressing the human elastin promoter/CAT reporter gene construct.
(A) CAT activity responds in a dose-dependent manner to UVB in mice. Single dose with energy fluencies indicated increased CAT activities up to 8.5-fold, as compared to irradiated control mice (0).
(B) Dermal fibroblasts derived from transgenic mice were exquisitely sensitive to UVB, with maximal promoter activation being more than 30-fold higher than non-irradiated control cultures (0) after a single dose of UVB of only 5.5 mJ/cm^2. **(C)** CAT activity increased in response to UVA in vivo. Single doses of 9.5 and 38.2 J/cm^2 of UVA increased CAT activity less than 2-fold over non-irradiated controls (0). **(D)** UVA irradiation failed to increase CAT activity in vitro. Bars indicate mean ± SD (adapted from [19]).

efficient in enhancing elastin promoter activity than UVA alone. For this purpose, PUVA was tested both *in vivo* and *in vitro* models based on the transgenic mouse line or cell cultures established from the skin of these animals [24]. In the *in vivo* model, the transgenic mice were topically treated with 8-MOP solution (2 mg/ml) and then subjected to UVA (10 J/cm^2). The control animals received either 8-MOP or UVA alone, or remained untreated. Treatment of the animals with 8-MOP alone resulted in 1.4-fold enhancement of the promoter activity, while 10 J/cm^2 UVA irradiation enhanced the activity by 1.7-fold. However, a combination of 8-MOP and UVA (PUVA) resulted in ~4-fold enhancement of the elastin promoter activity *(Fig. 5)*. These results were confirmed in *in vitro* PUVA experiments. In these studies, cell cultures were incubated with 1.0 μg/ml of 8-MOP and then subjected to 0.5, 0.75 or 1.0 J/cm^2 of UVA. Again, untreated cell cultures, or those receiving either 1.0 μg/ml of 8-MOP or 1.0 J/cm^2 of UVA alone, served as controls. Either 8-MOP or UVA alone resulted in minimal increases in elastin promoter activity, while a combination of both resulted in a UVA-concentration dependent enhancement of CAT activity. Specifically, UVA, in the presence of 0.5, 0.75 or 1.0 J/cm^2 resulted in 6.3, 13.4, and 18.0-fold enhancement of the elastin promoter activity, respectively *(Fig. 6)*.

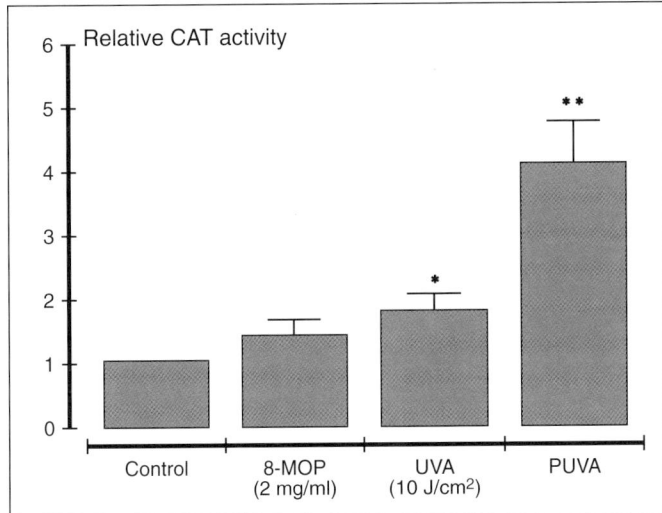

Figure 5. *Demonstration that PUVA treatment of transgenic mice increases CAT activity in vivo. Mice were pretreated topically with an ethanolic solution of 8-MOP (2 mg/ml) prior to irradiation with 10 J/cm^2 of UVA. The CAT activity increased over 3-fold in PUVA-treated mice (PUVA), as compared to untreated controls. Mice receiving 8-MOP alone (8-MOP) or UVA alone (UVA) demonstrated small alterations in CAT activity, as compared to controls. Bars indicate mean ± SEM (adapted from [24]).*

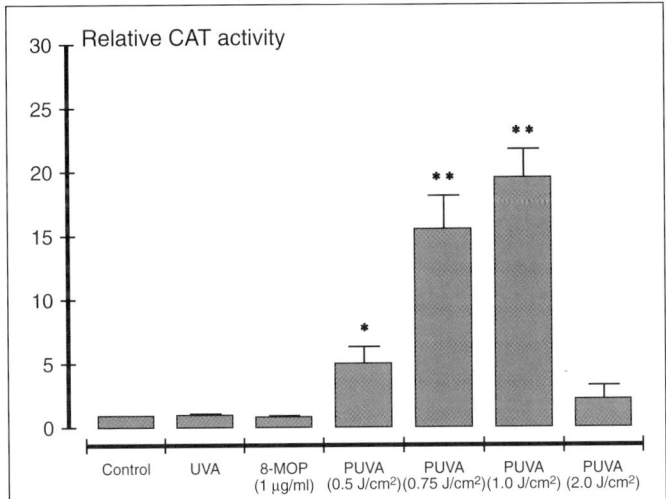

Figure 6. *Demonstration that PUVA treatment of cultured fibroblasts up-regulates elastin promoter activity. Fibroblasts derived from the skin of transgenic mice containing the human elastin promoter/CAT construct were preincubated with a concentration of 1 mg/ml of 8-MOP and then exposed to increasing amounts of UVA (PUVA). The UVA doses in J/cm^2 are shown in parentheses under each pair of samples. Statistical significance is indicated by asterisks : * $p < 0.05$; ** $p < 0.01$. Bars indicate mean ± SEM (adapted from [24]).*

Collectively, these results confirmed the role of UVB in elastin promoter activation in photoaging and they further identified UVA as a contributory factor *in vivo*. The differential effects of UVA and UVB may be due to the far greater ability of UVB to generate DNA photoproducts as compared to UVA. This possibility was supported by experiments utilizing PUVA, since addition of 8-MOP markedly increases the formation of photoproducts in DNA. This transgenic mouse model, therefore, serves as a useful system to study mechanisms of cutaneous photoaging, and it provides a convenient model to test compounds that may protect the skin against photodamage.

Acknowledgements

Tsunemichi Takeuchi and Sung Kong assisted in these studies. Carol Kelly provided excellent secretarial help. The original studies by the authors were supported by the United States Public Health Service, National Institutes of Health grant RO1-AR28450, and by the Dermatology Foundation.

References

1. Gilchrest BA. Skin aging and photoaging: an overview. *J Am Acad Dermatol* 1989; 21: 610-3.
2. Balin AK, Allen RG. Mechanisms of biologic aging. In: Gilchrest BA, ed. *Dermatologic clinics.* Philadelphia: WB Saunders Company, Chapter 1, 1986: 347-58.
3. Perejda AJ, Uitto J. Nonenzymatic glycosylation of collagen and other proteins: relationship to development of diabetic complications. *Collagen Rel Res* 1982; 2: 81-8.
4. Bernstein EF, Uitto J. The effect of photodamage on dermal extracellular matrix. *Clinics in Dermatology* 1996; 14: 143-51.
5. Uitto J, Matsuoka LY, Kornberg RL. Elastic fibers in cutaneous elastoses. In: Rudolph R, ed. *Problems in aesthetic surgery: biological causes and clinical solutions.* St. Louis: The CV Mosby Co., Chapter 15, 1986: 307-38.
6. Chen VL, Fleischmajer R, Schwartz E, Palia M, Timpl R. Immunochemistry of elastotic material in sun-damaged skin. *J Invest Dermatol* 1986; 87: 334-7.
7. Mera SL, Lovell CR, Jones RR, Davies JD. Elastic fibres in normal and sun-damaged skin: an immunohistochemical study. *Br J Dermatol* 1987; 117: 21-7.
8. Dahlback K, Ljungquist A, Lofberg H, Dahlback B, Engvall E, Sakai LY. Fibrillin immunoreactive fibers constitute a unique network in the human dermis: immunohistochemical comparison of the distributions of fibrillin, vitronectin, amyloid P component and orcein stainable structures in normal skin and elastosis. *J Invest Dermatol* 1990; 94: 284-91.
9. Bernstein EF, Underhill CP, Hahn PJ, Brown DB, Uitto J. Chronic sun-exposure alters both the content and distribution of dermal glycosaminoglycans. *Br J Dermatol* 1996; 135: 255-62.
10. Bernstein EF, Fisher LW, Li K, LeBaron RG, Tan EML, Uitto J. Differential expression of the versican and decorin genes in photoaged and sun-protected skin: comparison by immunohistochemical and Northern analyses. *Lab Invest* 1995; 72: 662-9.
11. Rosenbloom J. The elastic fiber in health and disease. In: Moshell AN, ed. *Dermatology foundation: progress in dermatology* 1996; 30: 1-15.
12. Uitto J. Molecular Pathology of Collagen. In: Abantangelo G, Davidson J, eds. *Cutaneous development, aging and repair.* Padova: Liviana Press, Fidia Research Series, 1989; 18: 9-29.
13. Bernstein EF, Chen YQ, Tamai K, Shepley KJ, Resnik KS, Zang H, Tuan R, Mauviel A, Uitto J. Enhanced elastin and fibrillin gene expression in chronically photodamaged skin. *J Invest Dermatol* 1994; 103: 182-6.
14. Johnston KJ, Oikarinen AI, Lowe NJ, Clark JG, Uitto J. Ultraviolet radiation-induced connective tissue changes in the skin of hairless mice. *J Invest Dermatol* 1984; 82: 587-90.
15. Kligman LH, Akin FJ, Kligman AM. The contributions of UVA and UVB to connective tissue damage in hairless mice. *J Invest Dermatol* 1985; 84: 272-6.
16. Bissett DL, Hannon DP, Orr TV. An animal model of solar-aged skin: histological, physical and visible changes in UV-irradiated hairless mouse skin. *Photochem Photobiol* 1987; 46: 367-76.
17. Bissett DL, Hannon DP, Orr TV. Wavelength dependence of histological, physical and visible changes in chronically UV-irradiated hairless mouse skin. *Photochem Photobiol* 1989; 50: 763-9.
18. Kligman L, Sayre R. An action spectrum for ultraviolet induced elastosis in hairless mice: quantification of elastosis by image analysis. *Photochem Photobiol* 1990; 53: 237-42.
19. Bernstein EF, Brown DB, Urbach F, Forbes D, Del Monaco M, Wu M, Katchman SD, Uitto J. Ultraviolet radiation activates the human elastin promoter in transgenic mice: a novel *in vivo* and *in vitro* model of cutaneous photoaging. *J Invest Dermatol* 1995; 105: 269-73.

20. Hsu-Wong S, Katchman S, Ledo I, Wu M, Khillan J, Bashir MM, Rosenbloom J, Uitto J. Tissue-specific and developmentally regulated expression of human elastin promoter activity in transgenic mice. *J Biol Chem* 1994; 269: 18072-5.
21. Katchman SD, Hsu-Wong S, Ledo I, Wu M, Uitto J. Transforming growth factor-b up-regulates human elastin promoter activity in transgenic mice. *Biochem Biophys Res Comm* 1994; 203: 485-90.
22. Reitamo S, Remitz A, Tamai K, Ledo I, Uitto J. Interleukin-10 up-regulates elastin gene expression *in vivo* and *in vitro* at the transcriptional level. *Biochem J* 1994; 302: 331-3.
23. Mauviel A, Chen YQ, Kähäri V-M, Ledo I, Wu M, Rudnicka L, Uitto J. Human recombinant interleukin-1b up-regulates elastin gene expression in dermal fibroblasts. Evidence for transcriptional regulation both *in vitro* and *in vivo*. *J Biol Chem* 1993; 268: 6520-4.
24. Bernstein EF, Gasparro FP, Brown DB, Takeuchi T, Kong SK, Uitto J. 8-methoxypsoralen and ultraviolet A radiation activate the human elastin promoter in transgenic mice: *in vivo* and *in vitro* evidence for gene induction. *Photochem Photobiol* 1996; 64: 369-74.

Effects of repeated suberythemal doses of UVA in human skin

S. Seité, D. Moyal, S. Richard, J. de Rigal, J.-L. Lévêque, C. Hourseau, A. Fourtanier

S. Seité, S. Richard, J.-L. Lévêque, A. Fourtanier: L'Oréal, Centre de Recherche Charles-Zviak, 90, rue du Général-Roguet, 92583 Clichy Cedex, France.
D. Moyal, C. Hourseau: L'Oréal, Centre Eugène-Schueller, 92117 Clichy Cedex, France.
J. de Rigal: L'Oréal, 1, avenue Eugène-Schueller, 93601 Aulnay-sous-Bois Cedex, France.

There is now evidence that UVA wavelengths (320-400 nm) in sunlight may contribute to the clinical changes commonly observed in photodamaged skin. We examined the effects of repetitive, suberythemal doses of UVA radiation on human skin in order to identify the epidermal and dermal changes indicative of early tissue injury. For these purpose, two areas of the back of fourteen female volunteers, phototype I to III, 20 to 40-year-old, were exposed three times a week for 13 weeks, to increasing doses of UVA (330-440 nm) resulting in a cumulative dose of 1,200 J/cm^2. During the exposure period, biophysical and clinical changes were examined. After the last irradiation, a series of epidermal and dermal parameters were analyzed and quantified by histochemical staining in combination with image analysis on biopsied tissue sections. UVA induced a strong pigmentation with no alteration of microtopography. Skin hydration and elasticity decreased, whereas total skin thickness, assessed by echography, remained unchanged. Histologically, irradiated epidermis revealed an absence of hyperplasia, a significant thickening of the stratum corneum with an increased number of stratum corneum layers, a depletion of Langerhans cells and an increase in the expression of the protective protein, ferritin. No significant alteration was seen using antisera against type IV collagen or laminin, suggesting that the dermal-epidermal junction (DEJ) was largely preserved. In the dermis, enhanced expression of tenascin was seen below the DEJ, but type I procollagen localized at the same site was unaltered. Although we were unable to visualize any change in elastic fiber content using Luna staining, using an immunofluorescence technique we noticed an increased deposition of lysozyme on elastin fibers, confirming the results of Lavker. These findings suggest that chronic suberythemogenic doses of UVA, resulted in morphological and histological skin changes.

There is now considerable evidence that UVA radiation may contribute to the clinical changes commonly observed in photodamaged skin. Animal studies have repeatedly shown that prolonged irradiation with UVA can induce non-melanoma skin cancer [1], inflammation [2] and significant connective tissue damage including elastosis, which is a prominent histological feature of photoaged skin [3, 4]. Furthermore, UVA may also contribute to the development of malignant melanoma [5].

More recently, Lavker *et al.* [6, 7] have identified histological and morphological changes that can serve as early markers of chronic UVA damage in human skin. They also studied the effects of daily exposure to relatively small suberythemogenic fluences of UVA (5-20 J/cm^2) for 8 days. They found histologically, epidermal hyperplasia, inflammation and deposition of lysozyme along the dermal elastic fiber network. It seems that UVA I (340-400 nm) was as effective as UVA I + II (320-400 nm). These changes were not prevented by a high SPF sunscreen containing 3% oxybenzone (UVB-UVA absorber) and 8% octyl dimethyl *p*-aminobenzoic acid (UVB absorber) [6]. Kligman *et al.* [8] have demonstrated the protective effect of a broad-spectrum sunscreen containing avobenzone (Parsol 1789, UVA I absorber) but not of one containing oxybenzone against histological and ultrastructural changes induced by chronic UVA I irradiation in hairless mice.

Lowe *et al.* [9] have determined the cutaneous effects of suberythemal and minimal erythemal doses of UVA in humans. They found, surprisingly, that both repeated suberythemal and erythemal UVA exposure produced a persistent reduction in elastic tissue content. This was observed after only 12 weeks of irradiation.

We examined the clinical, biophysical and histological changes produced in normal human skin by repeated exposures (13 weeks) to increasing low doses of UVA and some visible light (330-440 nm).

Materials and methods

Study population

Fourteen, healthy Caucasian females were enrolled after signing an informed consent that had been approved by a medical ethics committee. The volunteers were between 20 and 40 years old and of skin type I (2 subjects) II (6 subjects) and III (6 subjects). Skin of the untanned, mid-back region was the area chosen for exposure.

Experimental procedure

The source of UVA radiation was an UVASUN 5000 Lamp (Mutzhas, Munich, Germany) that we equipped with a Schott WG 335/3 mm filter and a black filter to obtain a spectrum between 330 and 440 nm *(Fig. 1)*. The spectral power distribution at the skin level was measured with a spectroradiometer, Macam 3010 (Macam, Scotland). The daily output was monitored with an Centra Osram UVmeter equipped with an UVA sensor. Two areas, (8 cm by 8 cm), were randomized and delimited with a template on the back. One area was not

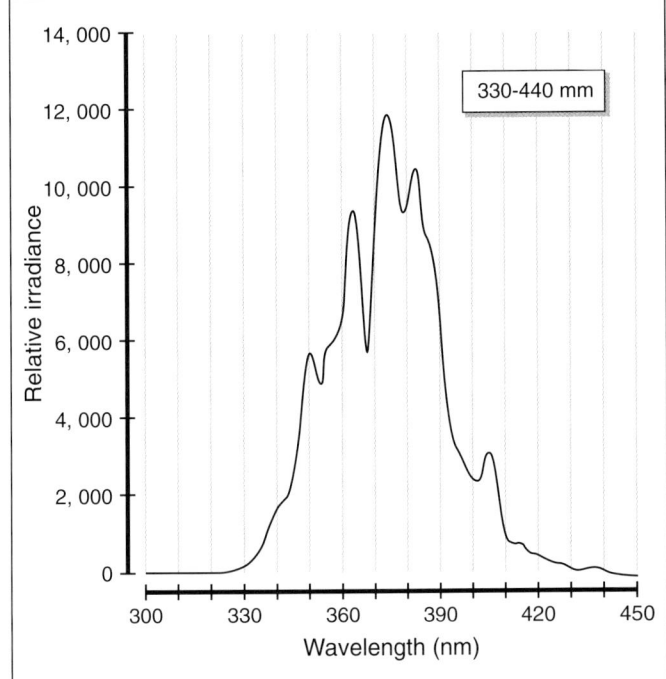

Figure 1. *Spectral distribution of UVASUN 5000 modified lamp equipped with WG335/3 mm and black filters. The spectrum was measured with a spectroradiometer Macam 3010.*

irradiated (–UVA) and the second was irradiated (+UVA) three times a week (Monday, Wednesday and Friday) for 13 weeks. The repeated dosing schedule was chosen to be progressive and realistic. The UVA dose was increased (20% progression) each week according to the *Table I*. The total UVA dose received was 1,237 J/cm².

Biophysical assessments

Biophysical assessments were conducted before the first exposure : and during the exposure period at weeks 3, 6, 8, 10 and 12. Skin thickness was measured using an ultrasound echographic method (L'Oréal). The mode A echograph was equipped with a 25 MHz giving a resolution of 60.7 µm. The results were the mean of 2 determinations for each zone. Biome-

Table I. *Daily doses for UVA exposure schedule*													
Week	1	2	3	4	5	6	7	8	9	10	11	12	13
UVA dose (J/cm2)	10	12	14.4	17.3	20.8	25	30	36	43.2	51.8	51.8	51.8	51.8

18 J/cm² of UVA are equal to about 1 h sunshine on the French riviera at noon.
25 J/cm² are equal to about 0.5 MED of UVA for a phototype II to III person.
The total UVA dose delivered was 1,237 J/cm2.

chanical properties were assessed using a Twistometer® (L'Oréal). The elasticity (Ur/Ue) of the epidermis was determined. Skin hydration was measured using a Dermodiag® (L'Oréal) which determines electrical conductance at 10 MHz. Six measurements per area were performed and the mean calculated.

Microtopography – skin replica

Skin replicas were made using a silicon polymer before the first exposure on each area and then at weeks 3, 6, 8, 10 and 12 at the same location. These replicas were evaluated by computer image analysis. A number of parameters can be computed including the line densities of the furrows and their average depth and the coefficient of developed skin surface (CDSS) which is the mathematical expression of true *versus* apparent surface area.

Skin pigmentation

Skin pigmentation was determined each week using a CR200 Chromameter (Minolta). Results were expressed as the mean of 4 measurements.

Biopsy specimen – histological and immunofluorescence evaluations

Four days after the last exposure, a 4 mm punch biopsy specimen was obtained from each area. Biopsies were immediately placed in liquid nitrogen and kept at – 80° C until use. Frozen skin samples were embedded in Tissue-Tek® (Miles, USA) and cut into 5 µm, vertical cryostat sections. For histological studies, sections were fixed in 10% buffered formalin and processed for light microscopy. Haematoxylin-phloxin-saffran (HPS) was used for overall morphologic evaluation by a pathologist and measurements of the stratum corneum and viable epidermal thickness were performed with a computerized image analyser ASM68K (Leica, France). The number of stratum corneum layers was also determined on methylene blue-stained 5 µm cryostat sections after incubation with 0.5 N NaOH (Prolabo, France). Paraffin sections were stained with Luna's aldehyde fuchsin as well as with orcein for the visualization and the quantification of elastic fibers, Mowry's combined with Van Gieson's stain for glycosaminoglycan deposition (GAG), and Fontana Masson for melanization. Elastic tissue content was quantified with a computer-assisted, color image analysis system (Leica, France). All samples were quantified by the same operator and the elastic tissue content was expressed as a percentage of the overall dermal area examined.

For indirect immunofluorescence microscopy, cryostat sections were air dried, rinsed in phosphate buffered saline (PBS), pH7.2 (Biomérieux Laboratories, France) and immunolabeled at room temperature with antisera diluted in PBS as follow: 1/10, 1/20 and 1/160 for rabbit antisera against human type I, III and IV collagens (IPL France), 1/30 for rabbit antiserum against human fibronectin and 1/50 for guinea pig antiserum against human elastin (IPL, France), 1/160 for rabbit antiserum against mice laminin (IPL, France), 1/200 for rat anti-human pro-collagen I amino-terminal monoclonal antibody (Chemicon, USA), 1/1,000 for rabbit antiserum against human ferritin (Sigma, France) and 1/10 for rabbit antisera against human tenascin (Life Technologies, France). Rabbit antisera against human alpha-1 antitrypsin (Immunon, USA) or against lysozyme (Zymed, USA) were used undiluted. Sections were incubated with each antibody for 60 min at room temperature or overnight at 4° C, washed with PBS, incubated with fluorescein isothiocyanate (FITC) conjugated goat anti-rabbit IgG or Rhodamine (TRITC) conjugated swine anti-guinea pig IgG from Dako (Denmark) (dilution 1/50) for 60 min, washed again with PBS, incubated with propidium iodide 1/10 for nucleus staining, washed with PBS and mounted. Fluorescence was evaluated using a four-point scoring scale: 1, mild; 2, moderate; 3, intense; and 4, very intense fluorescence.

Stastistical analysis

Statistical analyses were performed with an analysis of variance model (SAS, PROC GLM) including factors for subjects, treatment and time.

Results

Clinical and biophysical data

For the microtopography, the 3 parameters examined (number, depth of furrows and CDSS) were not significantly modified by the UVA exposures. The epidermal elasticity was expressed in relative unit *versus* the value obtained before the first irradiation because there was an effect of the location of the sites on the back. A decrease of 15 to 20% of epidermal elasticity was observed on the irradiated site *(Fig. 2)*.

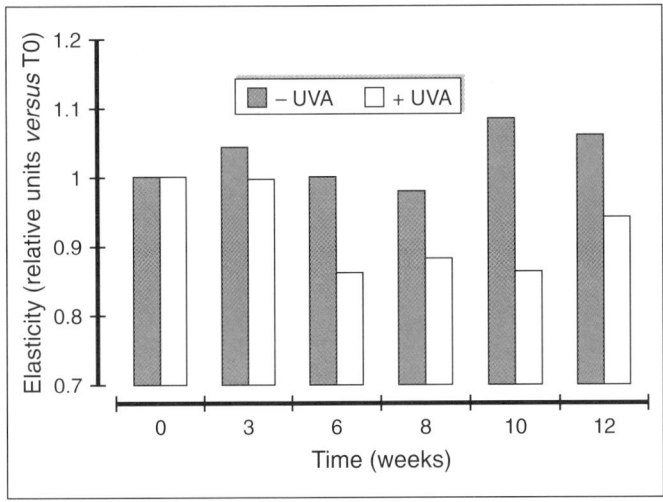

Figure 2. *Effect of UVA on epidermal elasticity (Ur/Ue). A decrease of 15-20% of epidermal elasticity was noted at the UVA irradiated site.*

The conductance, which reflects the degree of hydration of the stratum corneum, was decreased in the exposed area *(Fig. 3)*.

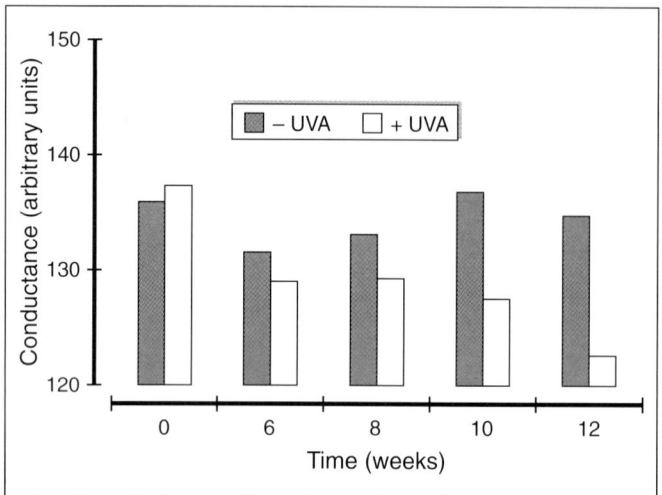

Figure 3. *Effect of UVA on skin hydration. The conductance decreased at the exposed site.*

Before and after exposure, the total skin thickness, assessed by echographic measurements, was similar (2.4 ± 0.1 mm) on the two areas.

Clinically, no erythema was detected throughout the entire period of exposure. The pigmentation evaluated by the luminance parameter (L) increased strongly on the area exposed to UVA. This result was confirmed by histological examination after Fontana Masson staining.

Histology and immunofluorescence

- *Epidermis.* In assessing the effects of UVA irradiation on the epidermis, the change in thickness of the viable epidermis (basal, spinous and granular layers) was evaluated separately from the stratum corneum. These quantitative results are presented in the *Table II*. UVA exposures induced a non-significant epidermal hyperplasia associated with a significant ($p \leq 0.05$) thicke-

Table II. *Morphological changes after repeated UVA exposures*		
Parameter	Non-irradiated (n = 14)	UVA (n = 14)
Stratum corneum thickness (mm)	16.41 ± 1.33	19.05 ± 0.97
Stratum corneum layers (number)	11.61 ± 0.45	14.69 ± 0.86*
Viable epidermal thickness (mm)	72.53 ± 4.48	75.74 ± 6.02
Elastic fiber quantification (%)	20.01 ± 1.24	20.42 ± 1.20
Tenascin deposition (visual assessment)	1.36 ± 0.21	2.79 ± 0.24*

* $p \leq 0.05$ compared to the non-irradiated area.

ning of the stratum corneum and an increase of the number of stratum corneum layers. Apart from changes in thickness and a prominent deposition of melanin, the epidermis did not appear to be morphologically altered at the irradiated site. No sunburn cells (SBC) were detected.

In non-exposed sites, ferritin was detected principally in the basal keratinocyte layer of the epidermis. UVA exposure induced an increased expression of ferritin in the basal and suprabasal epidermal layers and in interstitial dermal cells *(Fig. 4)*.

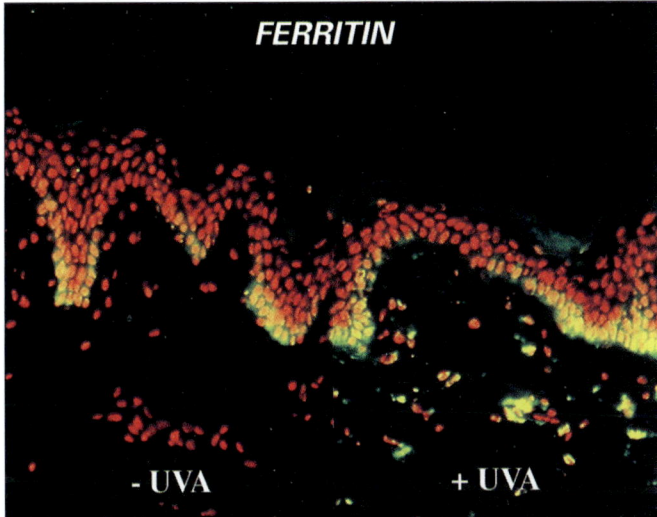

Figure 4. *Effect of UVA on ferritin expression in human skin. Immunohistochemical demonstration showing increasing ferritin staining in basal and suprabasal keratinocyte layers and dermal interstitial cells in the UVA irradiated site.*

• *Dermis.* No marked dermal inflammation was noted after UVA exposure. No clear alteration of the dermal-epidermal junction (DEJ) was seen with the antisera directed against human type IV collagen or laminin. In 8 subjects, UVA irradiation induced a slight increase of blue-staining material identified as GAG. The most prominent dermal change was a marked increase of tenascin deposition below the DEJ *(Fig. 5)*. Type I pro-collagen localized at the same site was unaltered (data not shown). No modification of the fluorescence staining pattern was seen with the antisera directed against human type I and III collagens or fibronectin.

In Luna or Orcein stained sections, for 6 subjects elastic fibers were not markedly modified by UVA irradiation. For 5 subjects UVA induced a moderate elastic fiber hyperplasia. In 2 subjects the elastic fibers were slightly fragmented and in 1 subject they were thin and sparse. Image analysis quantification, based upon elastic tissue-like staining, showed no modification in elastic tissue content ($\approx 20 \pm 1\%$ of the dermis area examined in unexposed and exposed sites). This result was supported by the unmodified staining pattern observed in the two areas by indirect immunofluorescence with a specific antibody directed against human elastin *(Fig. 6)*. The dermal distribution pattern of the reaction products for lysozyme or alpha-1 antitrypsin were restricted to the elastin fiber network for lysozyme and to elastin fibers and a DEJ component for alpha-1 antitrypsin *(Figs. 6 and 7)*. UVA induced a significant increase in the depositions of lysozyme or alpha-1 antitrypsin in the dermis.

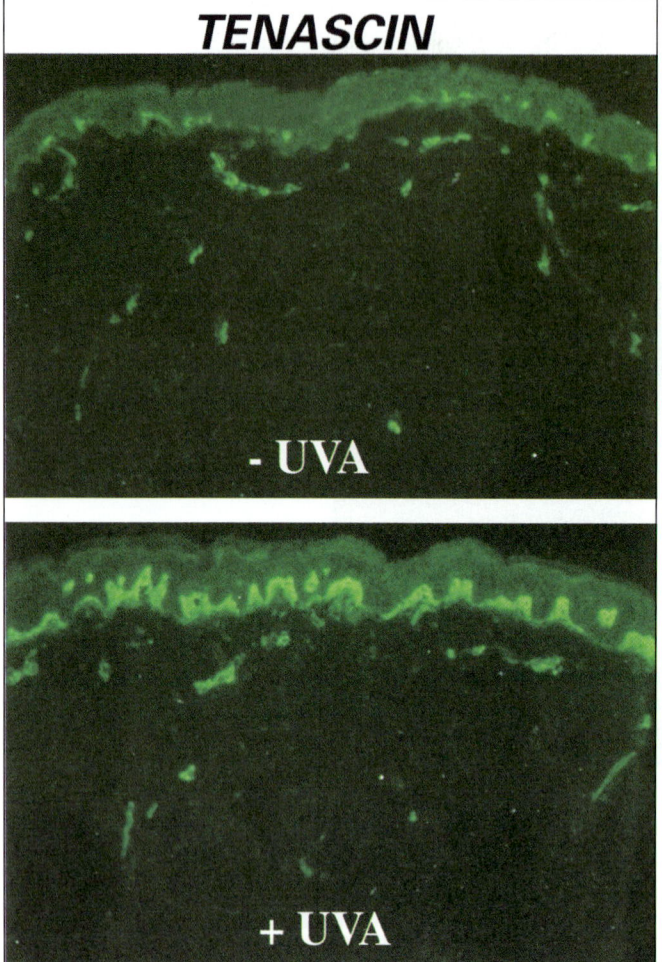

Figure 5. *Effect of UVA on tenascin expression in human skin. Immunohistochemical demonstration showing enhanced deposition of tenascin below the DEJ in the UVA irradiated site.*

Discussion

This present study confirms that repetitive UVA exposure of human skin results in some epidermal and dermal changes. Previous investigations on the effects of repetitive UVA irradiation in humans [6-9] have been performed in areas not previously exposed to sunlight (buttock) and was conducted with a xenon arc solar simulator delivering much more UVA II than the UVASUN lamp used in this study. The daily dose was also greater than in our experiment. In these other studies, authors noted an important erythemal response not seen with our protocol. These facts explain the more pronounced changes described in these manuscripts, such as epidermal hyperplasia, stratum corneum thickening and the presence of SBC or dermal inflammatory infiltrates.

Iron has been shown to be an important catalyst of reactive oxygen species reactions [10]. Chelation of intracellular iron with exogenous chelators or increased levels of endogenous

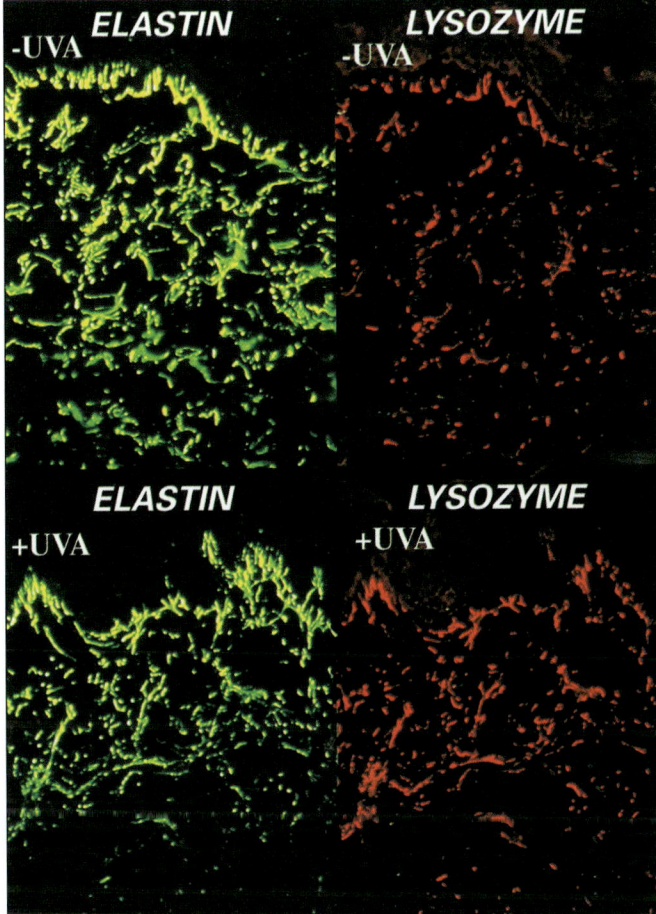

Figure 6. *Effect of UVA on elastin and lysozyme expression in human skin. Double immunostaining showing no alteration of the elastin staining pattern and sparse lysozyme deposition in non-irradiated dermis compared to prominent deposition on elastin fibers in the UVA irradiated dermis.*

iron storage protein, ferritin has been reported to protect mammalian cells from the damaging effects of oxidative stress generated by UVA radiation in particular [11]. Basal ferritin expression was relatively high in the basal keratinocytes of epidermis in an unexposed area (back skin). We have found that chronic UVA irradiation induced an enhanced expression of ferritin in basal and suprabasal epidermal layers and in interstitial dermal cells as described by Applegate *et al.* [12]. Increasing amounts of ferritin which indicate oxidative damage, would result in an enhancement of the cellular iron sequestering capacity and perhaps confer increased resistance to further oxidative stress. So, this protein may be considered as a good UVA marker.

In UVA irradiated areas, there was a marked deposition of lysozyme and alpha-1 antitrypsin. Lysozyme, an enzyme secreted by the monocytes-macrophages series and some epithelial cells, has been shown to be associated with damaged elastic fibers in many tissues. In skin, lysozyme is associated with elastic fibers in sun-damaged regions, and the number of lysozyme-containing elastic fibers appears to correlate with the amount of sun-damage [13, 14]. Recently Lavker *et al.* [6, 7] found that suberythemal doses of UVA produced a marked

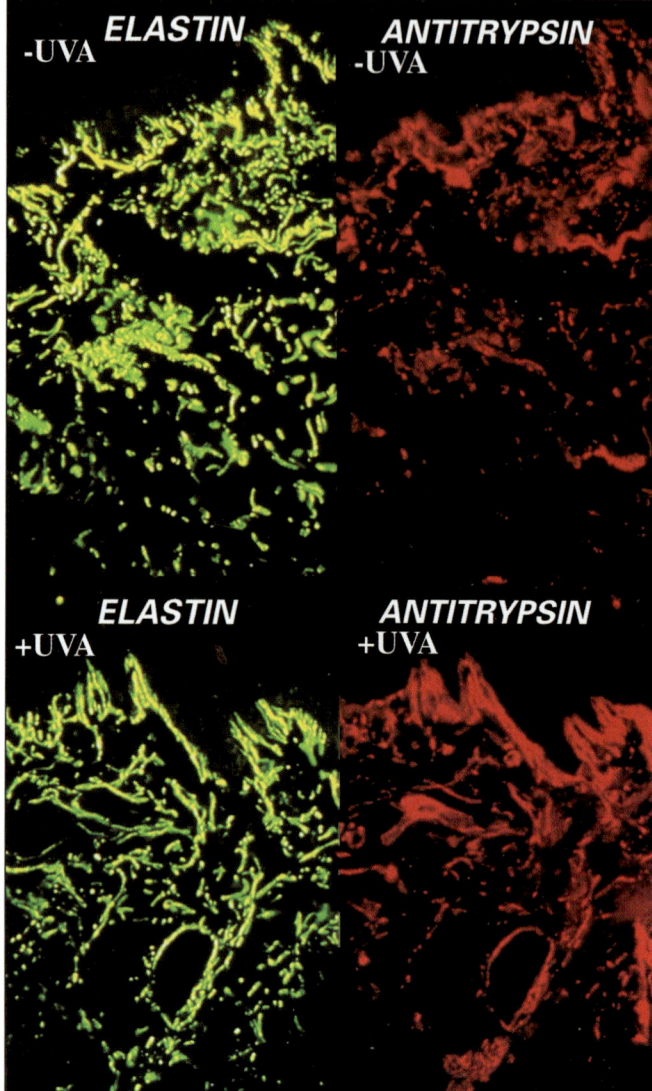

Figure 7. Effect of UVA on elastin and alpha-1 antitrypsin expression in human skin. Double immunostaining showing no alteration of the elastin staining pattern and a low alpha-1 antitrypsin deposition in non-irradiated dermis compared to the significant deposition on elastin fibers and a DEJ component in the UVA irradiated dermis.

increase in lysozyme deposition on elastic fibers in exposed skin. Park et al. [15] showed that lysozyme binds to the elastin component of elastic fibers; in so doing, lysozyme protects elastin from proteolytic degradation by elastases. In the same manner, alpha-1 antitrypsin, a major antiproteinase, which neutralizes multiple proteolytic enzymes ranging from collagenases to elastases, has been shown to be deficient in a number of inflammatory or immune-mediated diseases [16, 17].

These phenomena may be early events leading to solar elastosis associated with severe, sun damaged skin and perhaps may explain the decrease in epidermal elasticity.

Tenascin, is a large glycoprotein of the extracellular matrix, interacting with collagens, proteoglycans and fibronectin. This protein is secreted by dermal fibroblasts and also epidermal keratinocytes in culture [18] and is expressed at low levels in normal skin. Tenascin is upregulated in skin tumors, in a number of skin diseases with epidermal hyperproliferation and during wound healing [19, 20]. Suberythemal, low doses of UVA induced a significant increase of tenascin deposition below the DEJ, suggesting that tenascin-like lysozyme or alpha-1 antitrypsin may be viewed as early markers of UVA-induced dermal changes.

These results show that daily UVA photoprotection is needed to prevent alterations leading to photoaging and eventually skin cancers.

Acknowledgements

The authors wish to thank Dr. Flechet and Mrs Medaisko for the biopsy sampling of the volunteers, Mrs Tison, Lombard and Verdier for histological procedures, Mrs Charles for statistical evaluations and Mrs Olivry and Renault for technical and secretary assistance.

References

1. Van Weelden H, De Gruijl FR, Van der Leun JC. Carcinogenesis by UVA, with an attempt to assess the carcinogenic risks of tanning with UVA and UVB. In: Urbach F, ed. The biologic effects of UVA radiation. New York: Praeger, 1986: 137-46.
2. Lavker RM, Kligman AM. Chronic heliodermatitis: a morphologic evaluation of chronic actinic damage with emphasis on the role of mast cells. J Invest Dermatol 1988; 90. 325-30.
3. Kligman LH, Akin FJ, Kligman AM. The contribution of UVA and UVB to connective tissue damage in hairless mice. J Invest Dermatol 1985; 84: 272-6.
4. Gilchrest BA. Skin aging and photoaging: an overview. J Am Acad Dermatol 1989; 21: 610-3.
5. Setlow RB, Grist E, Thompson K, Woodhead AD. Wavelengths effective in induction of malignant melanoma. Proc Natl Acad Sci USA 1993; 90: 6666-70.
6. Lavker RM, Gerberick GF, Veres DA, Irwin CJ, Kaidbey KH. Cumulative effects from repeated exposures to suberythemal doses of UVB and UVA in human skin. J Am Acad Dermatol 1995; 32: 53-62.
7. Lavker RM, Veres DA, Irwin CJ, Kaidbey KH. Quantitative assessment of cumulative damage from repetitive exposures to suberythemogenic doses of UVA in human skin. Photochem Photobiol 1995; 62: 348-52.
8. Kligman LH, Zheng P. The protective effect of broad spectrum sunscreen against chronic UVA radiation in hairless mice: a histologic and ultrastructural assessment. J Soc Cosmet Chem 1994; 45: 21-33.
9. Lowe NJ, Meyers DP, Wieder JM, Luftman D, Borget T, Lehman MD, Johnson AW, Scott IR. Low doses of repetitive ultraviolet A induce morphologic changes in human skin. J Invest Dermatol 1995; 105: 739-43.
10. Halliwell B, Gutteridge JMC. Role of iron in oxygen radical reactions. Methods Enzymol 1984; 100: 47-56.
11. Vile GF, Tyrell RM. Oxidative stress resulting from ultraviolet A irradiation of human skin fibroblasts leads to a heme oxygenase-dependent increase in ferritin. J Biol Chem 1993; 268: 14678-81.
12. Applegate LA, Scaletta C, Fourtanier A, Mascotto RE, Frenk E. Expression of DNA damage and stress proteins by UVA radiation of human skin in vivo. 12th ICP, Vienna, 1996.

13. Mera SL, Lovell CR, Russel Jones R, Davies JD. Elastic fibres in normal and sun-damaged skin: an immunohistochemical study. Br J Dermatol 1987; 117: 21-7.
14. Albrecht S, Kahn HJ. Lysozyme in abnormal elastic fibers of cutaneous aging, solar elastosis, and pseudoxanthoma elasticum. J Cutan Pathol 1991; 18: 75-80.
15. Park PW, Biedermann K, Mecham L, Bissett DL, Mecham RP. Lysozyme binds to elastin and protects elastin from elastase-mediated degradation. J Invest Dermatol 1996; 106: 1075-80.
16. Hwang ST, Williams ML, McCalmont TH, Frieden IJ. Sweet's syndrome leading to acquired cutis laxa in an infant with alpha-1 antitrypsin deficiency. Arch Dermatol 1995; 131: 1175-7.
17. Heng MC, Allen SG, Kim A, Lieberman J. Alpha-1 antitrypsin deficiency in a patient with widespread prurigo nodularis. Australas J Dermatol 1991; 32: 151-7.
18. Latijnhouwers M, Bergers M, Ponec M, Dijkman H, Andriessen M, Schalkwijk J. Epidermal keratinocytes are a source of tenascin. XVth FECTS Meeting, Munich, 1996.
19. Lightner VA, Gumkowski F, Bigner DD, Erickson HP. Tenascin/hexabrachion in human skin: biochemical identification and localization by light and electron microscopy. J Cell Biol 1989; 108: 2483-93.
20. Schalkwijk J, Van Vlijmen I, Oosterling B. Tenascin expression in hyperproliferative skin diseases. Br J Dermatol 1991; 124: 13-20.

Protection of the Skin against Ultraviolet Radiations
A. Rougier, H. Schaefer, eds. John Libbey Eurotext, Paris © 1998, pp. 59-71

Effects of repeated low doses of solar simulated UVR in human. Comparison with severe photodamaged skin

S. Séité, S. Tison-Régnier, F. Christiaens, M.-P. Verdier, P. Piquemal, C. Montastier, A. Fourtanier

S. Seité, S. Tison-Régnier, F. Christiaens, M.-P. Verdier, A. Fourtanier: L'Oréal, Centre de Recherche Charles-Zviak, 90, rue du Général-Roguet, 92583 Clichy Cedex, France.

The aging process of the skin encompasses two clinically and biologically independent processes that occur simultaneously: chronological or intrinsic aging which affects skin by slow and irreversible degeneration of tissue, and extrinsic aging or photoaging which results from exposure to environmental factors including primarily ultraviolet radiation. In areas exposed to sun, skin damages resulting from photoaging are surimposed on tissue degeneration resulting from chronological aging. Chronological aging alone as seen in sun protected sites, leads to remarkably few clinically apparent changes. In contrast, photoaging leads to marked cutaneous changes characterized clinically by wrinkles, roughness, sallowness, mottled dyspigmentation, telangectasia and a variety of benign and malignant neoplasms [1]. Such as clinical contrast is mirrored in the microtopography of exposed versus protected aged skin.

Histological and ultrastructural studies have shown that changes in photoaged skin are found mainly in dermal connective tissue [2, 3]. The extracellular matrix in the dermis is composed primarily of type I collagen, with lesser amount of type III collagen, elastin, proteoglycans and fibronectin. Sun-exposed sites usually display loss of mature type I collagen with an increase in the collagen III/collagen I ratio. A significant correlation was found between reduced levels of type I collagen and the severity of photodamage in human skin [4]. The histopathological hallmark of photoaging is a massive accumulation of elastotic material in the upper and middle dermis [5]. This phenomenon, known as solar elastosis, has been ascribed to changes in elastin, the principal component of elastic fibers, because the accumulated material is identified with elastin-specific histologic stains. The accumulation of elastotic material is accompanied by degeneration of the surrounding collagen meshwork [6]. Sun-damaged skin is illustrated by the appearance of the neck in persons spending a lot of time outdoors without protective clothing or sunscreen. This phenomenon, termed "cutis rhomboidalis" nuchae, is characterized by skin that is leathery, inelastic and yellowish due to solar elastosis.

In order to understand the chronology of photoaging process and to modelize this complex phenomenon we compared the cutaneous changes induced by 6 weeks exposure to low doses of solar simulated radiation (SSR) in young volunteers to those of unexposed and exposed aged skin ("cutis rhomboidalis" nuchae).

Experimental details

Study population

Healthy caucasian volunteers were enrolled after signing an informed consent that was approved by a medical ethics committee. The first group (group I) of ten volunteers were 52 to 71 years old with skin type III and IV, used to spend 6 hours average per day outdoor. These volunteers presented a typical photoaged neck skin clinically diagnosed as "cutis rhomboidalis" nuchae. They were also selected on the basis of a clear delineation between sun exposed and unexposed regions of the neck . The second group (group II) of twelve volunteers were 20 to 35 years old with skin type II and III. The untanned buttock region was used as the site for exposure.

UV source and dosimetry

SSR radiation source was an Oriel® 1000W xenon arc solar simulator equipped with a Schott® WG 320/2 mm filter and two step plates to deliver a solar simulating spectrum. The spectral power distribution at the skin level (40 cm from the lamp) was measured with a calibrated spectroradiometer (Macam 3010, Scotland) *(Figure 1)*. The daily output was monitored with a Centra Osram (Germany) UVmeter equipped with UVA and UVB sensors.

Exposure regimen

Two areas were delineated with a template on the buttock of group II volunteers. One area received no exposure (unexposed) and the second was exposed 5 days per week for 6 weeks (SSR exposed), to one individual minimal erythemal dose (MED) of SSR per exposure, which averaged 0.86 J/cm^2 UVB and 11 J/cm^2 UVA.

Clinical assessments and skin pigmentation

Clinical assessments were conducted on sun-exposed and unexposed areas of the neck for group I. For group II they were performed before, during and after exposure and skin pigmentation was assessed each week using a CR200 chromameter (Minolta, Japan). Results were expressed as the mean of 4 multiple measurements. The computerized chromameter calculated the trichromatic coordinates in the Lab C.I.E. 1976 system: illuminating C. The L^*, a^* and b^* coordinates were recorded and the individual typological angle (ITA = arc tangent $(L^*-50)/b^*$) calculated.

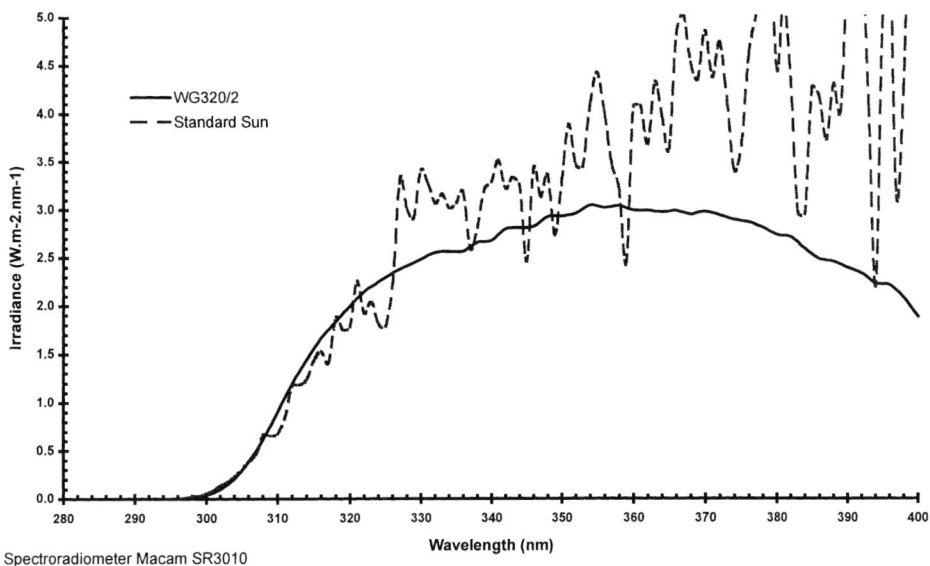

Figure 1. *Spectral power distribution at skin level of the radiations emitted from the filtered Xenon arc solar simulator. Spectrum was measured with a spectroradiometer Macam 3010. Relative irradiance is expressed in W / ($m^2.nm^{-1}$). Standard sun (DIN 67501) was multiplied by 5; so the slopes of the two spectra match in the UVB range.*

Skin microtopography

Using a computer image analysis system and an oblique illumination with an incident lighting angle of 26°, we measured the density of the furrows and their depth on silicone skin replicas obtained on unexposed and sun-exposed sites of group I of volunteers. Deep wrinkles are not taken in account when this lighting angle is used [11]. On volunteers of group II, skin microtopography was evaluated visually on skin replicas obtained on unexposed and SSR-exposed areas at day 0 and day 8 after the beginning of exposure, using an arbitrary 7 points grading scale (1 corresponding to just perceptible alteration and 7 to very severe changes).

Histology and immunohistochemistry

Biopsy samples were taken from unexposed and sun-exposed areas of group I volunteers and from unexposed and SSR-exposed areas (24 hours after last exposure) in group II volunteers. For histological studies, skin samples were fixed in 10% buffered formalin, embedded in paraffin and processed for light microscopy. Haematoxylin – phloxin – saffron (HPS) was used for overall morphological evaluation by a pathologist and measurement of viable epidermal thickness with a computerized image analyzer ASM68K (Leica, France). The number of stratum corneum layers was determined on methylene blue-stained 5 μm cryostat sections after incubation with 0.5N NaOH (Prolabo, France). Sections were also stained with Luna's aldehyde fuchsin as well as with orcein for visualization and quantification of elastic fibers.

For indirect immunofluorescence microscopy, cryostat sections were air dried, rinsed in phosphate buffered saline (PBS), pH 7.2 (Biomerieux Laboratories, France) and immunolabeled at room temperature with antisera diluted to PBS as follows: respectively 1/50 for guinea pig antiserum against human elastin (IPL, France), 1/200 for rat anti-human pro-collagen I amino-terminal monoclonal antibody (Chemicon, USA), 1/2000 for rabbit anti-bovine pro-collagen III amino-terminal polyclonal antibody (gift of Ch. Lapière, Liege, Belgium) and 1/10 for rabbit antiserum against human tenascin (Life Technologies, France). Rabbit antisera against human alpha-1 antitrypsin (Immunon, USA) or human lysozyme (Zymed, USA) were used undiluted. Cryostat sections were incubated with each antibody for 60 min. at room temperature or overnight at 4° C, washed with PBS, incubated with fluorescein isothiocyanate (FITC) conjugated goat anti-guinea pig or swine anti-rabbit IgG or rhodamine (TRITC) conjugated swine anti rabbit IgG from Dako (Denmark) (dilution 1/50 or 1/100) for 60 min., washed again with PBS, incubated with propidium iodide 1/10 for nucleus staining, washed with PBS and mounted.

Statistical analysis

Statistical analysis was performed using variance model (SAS, PROC GLM) including factors for subjects, treatments and times.

Results

Clinical aspects and skin pigmentation

For the two regions of the neck (sun-exposed/unexposed) of each subject of group I, a clinical score summing up individual grades for endpoints listed in *Table I* were given. Maximal score was 10 and minimal was 0. Average score on the 10 volunteers was 6.2 for sun-exposed area and 0 for unexposed area of the neck. Six over ten subjects were more pigmented in sun-exposed area. In group II, an erythema was detected on the SSR-exposed site in seven over twelve subjects after the first week of exposure and disappeared completely in all volunteers by the end of the fourth week of exposure.

Eleven subjects were pigmented after the first week and the last one after the second week of exposure. The pigmentation changes were evaluated by chromametry *(Table II)*. The measurements showed that ITA decreased steadily throughout the study. From light colour, the SSR-exposed areas turned to matt. Histological examination after Fontana Masson staining confirmed these observations. The deposition of melanin in SSR-exposed sites was more homogenous throughout epidermis than in group I sun-exposed sites *(Figure 2)*.

Table I. Clinical scoring for group I volunteers		
Endpoint	Clinical Assessment	Grade
Colour	Red brown Red Normal	2 1 0
Consistency	Flabby Lax Firm	2 1 0
Texture	Coarse Slight roughness Smooth	2 1 0
Sagging	Marked Moderate Slight	2 1 0
Wrinkling	Marked Moderate Slight	2 1 0

Clinical score: summing up (max. score = 10) of individual grades for each endpoint

Table II. Chromametry			
Group II relative variation# (n = 12)	Unexposed (%#)	SSR-exposed (%#)	Significance
ΔL^*	− 1	− 21.8	$p < 0.005$
Δb^*	4.1	39.2	$p < 0.005$
ΔITA	− 3.4	− 68	$p < 0.005$
Δa^*	7.8	134.2	$p < 0.005$

= (Day 43 − Day 1)/Day 1 values x 100.

Skin microtopography

Results from skin replicas analysis are presented in *Table III*. In sun-exposed regions of group I, the density of furrows was significantly reduced whereas their depth increased. For group II of volunteers changes as evaluated by visual assessment at the end of first week exposure, were similar to those observed in severe sun-damaged skin (group I) (decrease in number and increase in the depth of furrows) as mirrored by the mean of visual scores *(Table III)*.

Histology and immunohistochemistry

Morphometric examination of epidermis showed a significant thickening of the stratum corneum (SC) without change in the thickness of the viable epidermis (basal, spinous and granular layers) in exposed versus unexposed areas in both groups of volunteers *(Table IV)*.

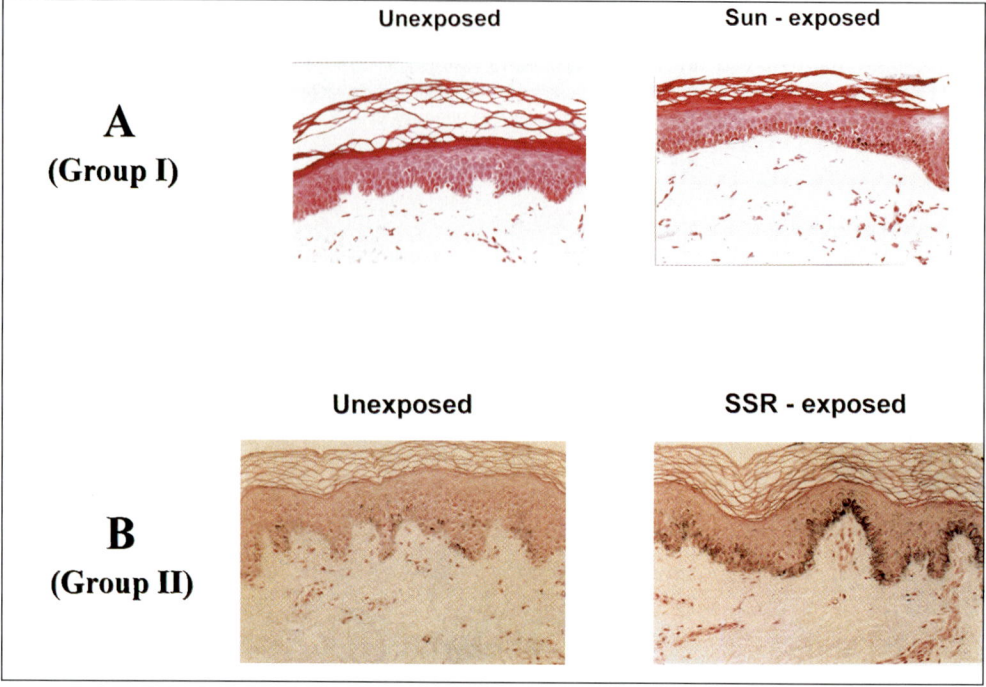

Figure 2. *Melanization - A: Group I: Sun-damaged and unexposed aged skin. B: Group II: SSR-exposed and unexposed skin (at day 43). Fontana Masson stain sections.*

Table III. ***Skin microtopography***			
Group I **Skin Furrows (n = 10)** (incident lighting angle: 26°)	**Unexposed**	**Sun-exposed**	**Significance**
Density per cm² Depth (μm)	37.0 ± 2.1 46.2 ± 7.3	26.2 ± 1.6 86.9 ± 9.5	$p < 0.001$ $p < 0.001$
Group II **Skin Furrows (n = 12)**	**Unexposed**	**SSR-exposed**	**Significance**
Visual score	0.04 ± 0.04	3.71 ± 0.44	$p < 0.001$

Results are mean ± SEM.

Table IV. ***Morphometry of the epidermis***			
Group I (n = 10)	**Unexposed**	**Sun-exposed**	**Significance**
Stratum corneum thickness (μm) Viable epidermis thickness (μm)	18.9 ± 2.1 71.2 ± 15.6	26.5 ± 4.0 72.3 ± 7.5	$p < 0.005$ NS
Group II (n = 12)	**Unexposed**	**SSR-exposed**	**Significance**
Stratum corneum layers number Viable epidermis thickness (μm)	14.6 ± 0.7 79.7 ± 3.5	20.6 ± 1.3 88.8 ± 1.7	$p < 0.005$ NS ($p = 0.005$)

Results are mean ± SEM. NS: Non Significant.

By immunohistochemistry, we studied various matrix components. Tenascin, a large glycoprotein, minimally expressed just below the dermal epidermal junction (DEJ) in normal skin, was slightly increased in the dermis and accumulated in the epidermis of sun-exposed skin samples *(Figure 3)*. This protein was significantly increased in the SSR-exposed skin biopsies but remained clearly located just below the DEJ *(Figure 3)*. Type I and III procollagens were predominantly in the extracellular papillary dermis as evidenced by immunohistochemistry. Relative staining intensities of type I and type III collagens were significantly altered in both cases. In sun-exposed biopsies, type I procollagen decreased whereas type III increased *(Figure 4)*. The same changes were observed in SSR-exposed biopsies with differences in staining intensity between the two groups of volunteers *(Figure 4)*. The decrease in type I procollagen staining pattern was higher after SSR exposure (group II) than in aged sun-exposed areas (group I). In contrast, the increased staining pattern of type III procollagen was lesser after SSR exposure (group II) than in aged sun-exposed areas (group I). Using a double staining technique, we looked simultaneously to elastin component of elastic fibers and to enzymes which have been described to be associated with damaged elastic fibers *e.g.* lysozyme and alpha-1 antitrypsin (7-8). As showed in *Figure 5* sun-aged skin biopsies (group I) presented severe elastosis. The dermal distribution patterns of reaction products or deposits from lysozyme or alpha-1 antitrypsin were restricted to the elastin fiber network and seemed to be correlated with the degree of photodamage. In contrast, six weeks of SSR-exposure were unable to induce any change into elastin network in group II subjects *(Figure 5)*. However lysozyme and alpha-1 antitrypsin deposits on elastin fibers were increased in SSR-exposed skin biopsies (group II) *(Figure 5)* but to a less extent than in sun-aged skin (group I). These depositions may be considered as an early events of solar elastosis process.

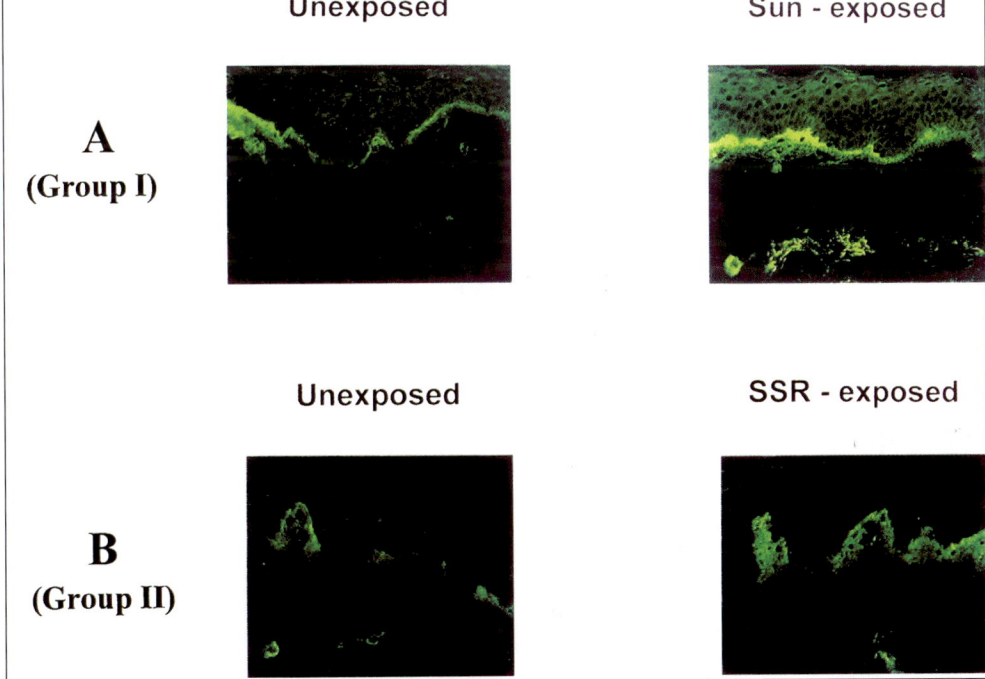

Figure 3. *Tenascin immunostaining. A: Group I: Sun-damaged and unexposed aged skin.*
B: Group II: SSR-exposed and unexposed skin.
Immunofluorescence microscopy using antiserum against human tenascin.

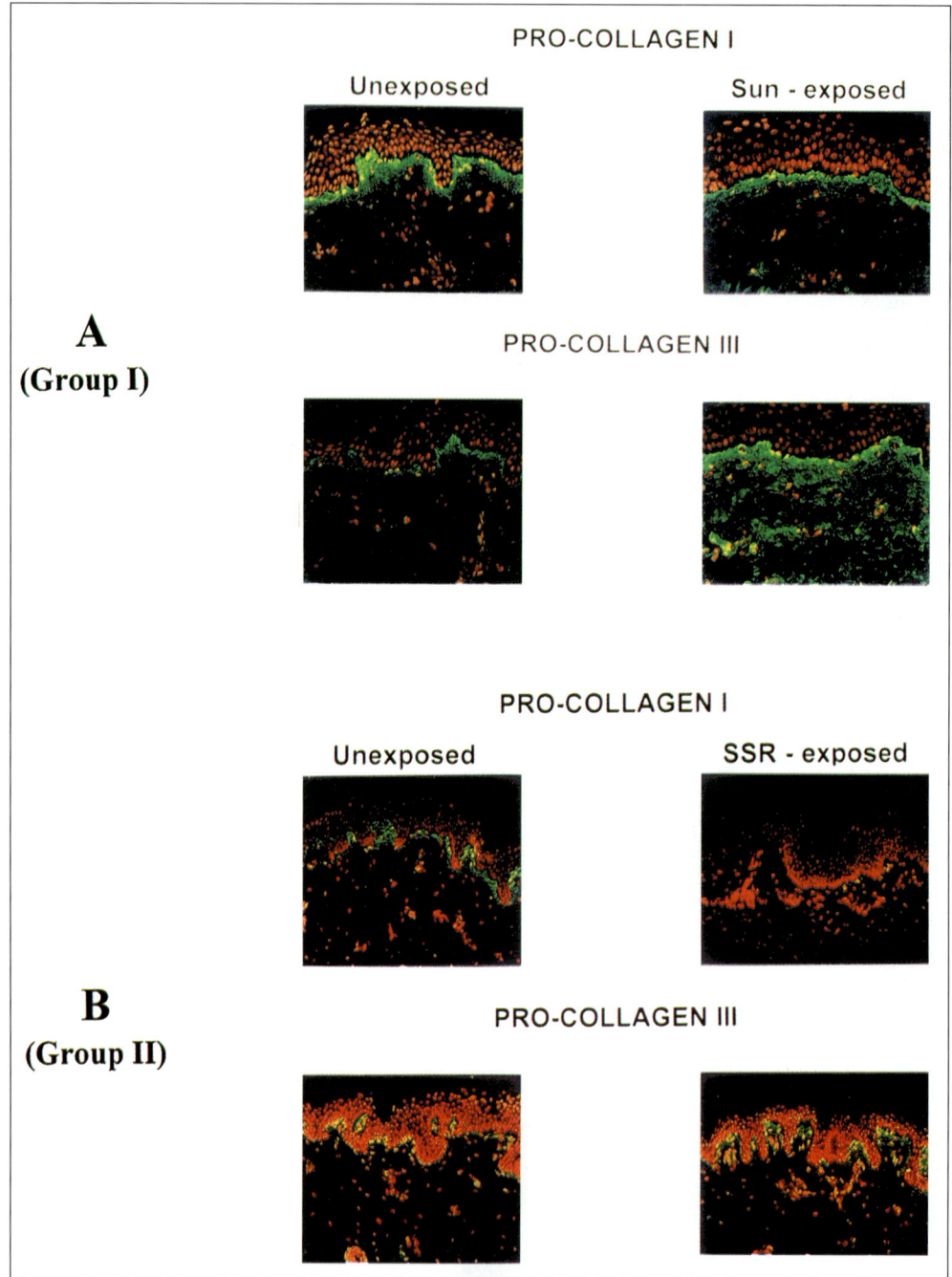

Figure 4. *Type I and III pro-collagens immunostaining.
A: Group I: Sun-damaged and unexposed aged skin. B: Group II: SSR-exposed and unexposed skin.
Immunofluorescence microscopy using antisera against human N-terminal
pro-collagen I or bovine N-terminal pro-collagen III.*

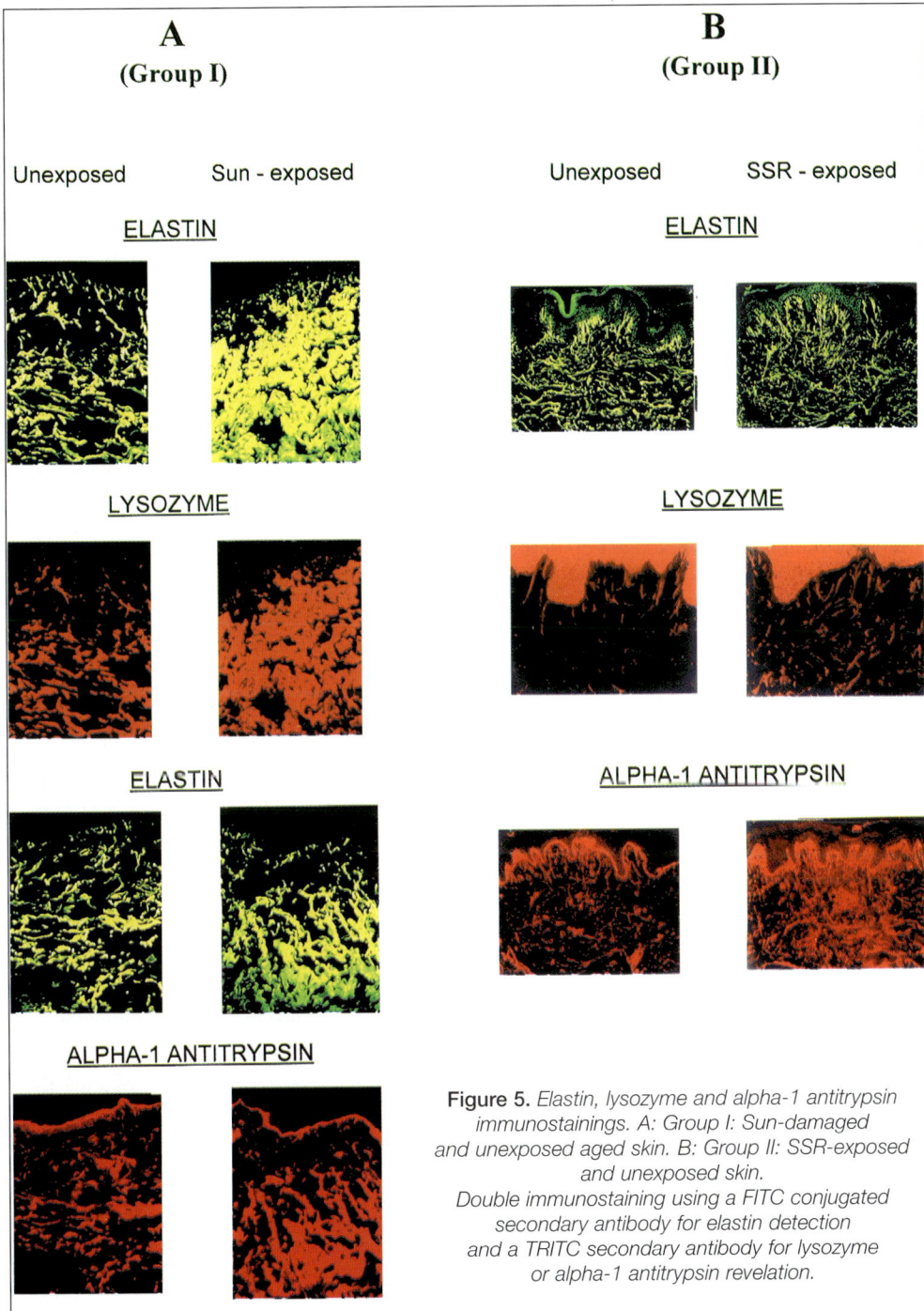

Figure 5. *Elastin, lysozyme and alpha-1 antitrypsin immunostainings. A: Group I: Sun-damaged and unexposed aged skin. B: Group II: SSR-exposed and unexposed skin. Double immunostaining using a FITC conjugated secondary antibody for elastin detection and a TRITC secondary antibody for lysozyme or alpha-1 antitrypsin revelation.*

Discussion

Chronic solar exposure is the major environmental insult that contributes to clinical and histological changes that we recognize as "aging" signs in sun-exposed skin areas (face, hands...) of an individual.

Reporting the results of a study on the side of the neck in people living or having lived for several years in Mediterranean areas, Adhoute et al (10) found a negative correlation between the degree of clinical elastosis and chromameter parameters L* (lightness) and b* (blue-yellow), as well as a positive correlation with the redness parameter a*. Multidimensional analysis of all parameters recorded in this experiment indicated that skin redness (reflecting inflammation or venous stasis) is most marked in subjects with severe elastosis [10]. In our study, each of the three parameters (L*, b*, a*) measured was significantly modified in SSR-exposed versus unexposed areas in the young volunteers of group II, but the most noticeable difference was seen for skin redness a* *(Table II)*.

One of the most striking clinical aspects of actinic aging is the heterogeneity of skin pigmentation which is clearly evidenced by the melanin distribution as observed after Fontana Masson staining. Variability in the degree of melanosome distribution within basal keratinocytes is another hallmark of photoaged epidermis [6]. Some keratinocytes appear sparsely melanized, while others contain abundant melanosomes, organized as a perinuclear cap. This contrasts with SSR-exposed keratinocytes where melanin appears more evenly distributed.

Compared with adjacent areas of the neck that are protected by clothing, the microrelief of photo-aged skin (group I) was deeper and less dense. These findings are in agreement with previous reports on skin microrelief in various areas of the body according to age [11]. It appears that both sun exposure and age lead to a deepening of skin furrows [12]. Repetitive exposure to 1 MED of SSR as well as a single dose exceeding MED [13] lead, a few days later, to changes in the microrelief similar to those seen in elderly people as illustrated by group II.

Photoaged epidermis is generally much thicker than either young or chronologically aged epidermis [14], but in the end stages of photodamage epidermal atrophy is noticed. Our results showed no clear modification of the viable epidermal thickness either in sun or SSR-exposed areas versus unexposed ones. In contrast a clear increase in stratum corneum thickness is shown in both group of volunteers. Generally few changes are noticeable in the organization of SC of photoaged versus protected site. However, somewhat more heterogeneity in SC organization and differences between sites of the body are seen in sundamaged skin areas [15].

Our immunohistological findings evidenced an increased staining with tenascin, a growth-modulating protein. In normal skin, the amount of tenascin is generally low and restricted to subepidermal areas and hair follicle [16]. However, in certain pathological conditions, such as skin tumors, hyperproliferative disorders and granulomatous skin diseases, there is a marked accumulation of tenascin in the dermis. In addition, during wound healing and healing blistering diseases large amounts of tenascin can be seen in the dermis. It is possible that the high level of tenascin observed in sun or SSR-exposed skin is non-specific. However, UVR is able to induce certain growth factors, such as TGF-β which has been shown to increase the deposition of tenascin [17]. It is interesting to note that though dermal tenascin expression increase in each group of volunteers, an increased epidermal expression is seen only in sun-exposed aged skin (group I).

Dermal damage induced by repetead UV irradiation is mainly reflected histologically e.g. by the disorganization of collagen fibrils [18] and accumulation of abnormal elastin-containing material [6]. These alterations are believed to be responsible for wrinkled appearance of sun-exposed skin. Biochemical evidence of connective-tissue alterations in photoaged skin includes reduced levels of type I and type III collagen precursors [19] and crosslinks [20], an increased ratio of type III to type I collagen [21] and an increased level of elastin. A significant correlation was found between reduced level of collagen type I and the severity of photodamage in human skin [4]. Our immunohistological results show a decreased type I and an increased type III procollagen expression principally located at the DEJ in all exposed skin samples. This location has been reported to be the site for new collagen synthesis [22].

The histologic hallmark of dermal photoaging is elastosis, a quantitative and qualitative change affecting elastic fibers. The magnitude of the progressive accumulation of elastic fibers is dependent on the degree of sun exposure [23]. Recent papers reporting an increased staining on abnormal elastic fibers from sun-damaged skin may provide some insights on the process of elastosis. Using immunohistochemical techniques, we and other investigators detected increasing lysozyme deposits on photodamaged elastic fibers, and the intensity of staining correlated positively with the extent of sun-damage [6-24]. Same phenomenon was observed for alpha-1 antitrypsin but the still unknown components of elastic fibers to which lysozyme or alpha-1 antitrypsin are bound seemed different (staining just below the DEJ for alpha-1 antitrypsin). Since lysozyme or alpha-1 antitrypsin at high concentration inhibits the activity of collagenase and elastase [25], It could be postulated that these proteins protect elastic fiber components from *in vivo* proteolysis [26]. Greater deposits of lysozyme or alpha-1 antitrypsin were found following SSR exposure. Since we were unable to detect any histological alteration in elastic fibers in SSR-exposed sites, an increase in these deposits may be viewed as an early marker for UVR-induced elastosis process.

All dermal proteins examined except elastin were modified in the same way in the two groups of volunteers. However some differences in staining intensities were observed as summarized in *Table V*. Tenascin and type I pro-collagen were more intensely changed in the SSR-exposed skin (group II) whereas type III pro-collagen, lysozyme and alpha-1 antitrypsin increased significantly more in sun-damaged aged skin (group I), which again suggests that tenascin and type I pro-collagen may be considered as early markers of photodamage whereas elastin and type III procollagen need longer exposure to be significantly impaired. Lysozyme and alpha-1 antitrypsin deposits appear early in sun-exposed skin and seem to be related to the severity of photodamage.

In conclusion, using repeated low doses of SSR for 6 weeks allows to reproduce most of the alterations observed in long term photoaging. The model may be used to evaluate the efficacy of products designed to prevent or repair skin damages induced by chronic sun exposure.

Table V. *Comparison of histological and immunohistochemical results of the two studies*		
Parameters	Sun-exposed	SSR-exposed (6 weeks)
Stratum corneum thickness	↗	↗
Viable epidermis thickness	Unchanged	Unchanged
Melanization	↗ (irregular)	↗ (homogeneous)
Tenascin (epidermis)	++	0
Tenascin (dermis)	↗	↗↗
Type I pro-collagen	↘	↘↘
Type III pro-collagen	↗↗	↗
Lysozyme	↗↗↗	↗
Alpha-1 antitrypsin	↗↗↗	↗
Elastin	↗↗↗	Unchanged

Acknowledgements

We thanks Dr. Spark and Dr. Stalder for biopsy sampling of the volunteers, Mrs. Lombard for histological procedures and Mrs. Charles for statistical evaluation.

References

1. Griffiths CEM. The clinical identification and quantification of photodamage. *Br J Dermatol* 1992; 127: 37-42.
2. Smith JG, Davidson EA, Sams WM, Clark RD. Alterations in human dermal connective tissue with age and chronic sun damage. *J Invest Dermatol* 1962; 39: 347-50.
3. Warren R, Garstein V, Kligman AM, Montagna W, Allendorf RA, Ridder GM. Age, sunlight and facial skin: a histologic and quantitative study. *J Am Acad Dermatol* 1991; 25: 751-60.
4. Yaar M, Gilchrest BA. Biochemical and molecular changes in photoaged skin. In: Gilchrest BA (ed.). *Photodamage*. Cambridge, New York, 1995: 168-84.
5. Kligman AM, Lavker RM. Heliodermatitis. In: Kligman AM, Takasy eds. *Cutaneous aging*. Tokyo: University of Tokyo press, 1988: 353-60.
6. Lavker RM. Cutaneous aging: Chronologic versus photoaging In Gilchrest BA, ed. *Photodamage*. Cambridge, Mass.: Blackwell Science 1995: 123-35.
7. Lavker RM, Kaidbey KH. The spectral dependence for UVA-induced cumulative damage in human skin. *J Invest Dermatol* 1997; 108: 17-21.
8. Seité S, Moyal D, Richard S, de Rigal J, Lévêque J, Hourseau C, Fourtanier A. Mexoryl SX: A broad absorption UVA filter protects human skin from the effects of repeated suberythemal doses of UVA. *J Photochem Photobiol* 1998; 44: 69-76.
9. Lever WF, Lever GS. Histopathology of the skin. Philadelphia: Lippincott. 249 (1975)
10. Adhoute H, de Rigal J, Marchand. JP, Privat Y. Lévêque JL. Influence of age and sun exposure on the biophysical properties of the human skin: an *in vivo* study. *Photodermatol Photoimmunol Photomed* 1992; 9: 99-103.
11. Corcuff P, Chatenay F, Lévêque JL. A fully automated system to study skin surface patterns. *Int J Cosmet Sci* 1984; 6: 167-76.
12. Lévêque JL. Non invasive measurements on photodamaged skin. In Gilchrest B.A., ed. *Photodamage*. Cambridge, Mass.: Blackwell Science, 1995: 185-200.
13. Pessis S, Grollier JF, Pasero R. Skin surface changes induced by UV irradiation. *Cosmet Technol Sci* 1982; 2: 293-310.
14. Kligman LH, Lavker RM. Cutaneous aging: The differences between intrinsic aging and photoaging. *J Cut Aging Cosmet Dermatol* 1988; 1: 5-11.
15. Bhadwan J, Chil-Hwan O, Lew R, Nehal KS, Labadie RR, Tsay A, Gilchrest BA. Histopathologic differences in the photoaging process in facial versus arm skin. *Am J Dermatopath* 1992; 14: 224-30.
16. Lightner VA, Gumkowski F, Bigner DD, Erickson HP. Tenascin/hexabrachion in human skin: Biochemical identification and localization by light and electron microscopy. *J Cell Biol* 1989; 108: 2483-93.
17. Pearson CA, Pearson D, Shibahara S. Tenascin cDNA cloning and induction by TGF-β. *Embo J* 1988; 7: 2977-82.
18. Bernstein EF, Chen YQ, Koop JB. Long-term sun exposure alters the collagen of the papillary dermis: Comparison of sun-protected and photoaged skin by northern analysis, immunohistochemical staining and confocal laser microscopy. *J Am Acad Dermatol* 1996; 34: 209-18.
19. Talwar HS, Griffiths CE, Fisher GJ, Hamilton TA, Voohrees JJ. Reduced type I and type III pro-collagens in photodamaged adult human skin. *J Invest Dermatol* 1990; 105: 285-90.
20. Yamauchi M, Prisavanh P, Haque Z, Woodley DT. Collagen cross-linking in sun-exposed and unexposed sites of aged human skin. *J Invest Dermatol* 1991; 97: 938-41.

21. Schwartz E, Cruickshank FA, Christensen CC, Perlish JS, Lebwohl M. Collagen alterations in chronically sun-damaged human skin. *Photochem Photobiol* 1993; 58: 841-4.
22. Fleischmajer R, Perlish JS, Timpl R. Collagen fibrillogenesis in human skin. *Ann Ny Acad Sci* 1985; 460: 246-57.
23. O'Brian JP, Regan W. A study of elastic tissue and actinic radiation in "aging", temporal arteries, polymyalgia, rheumatica and artherosclerosis. *J Am Acad Dermatol* 1991; 24: 765-76.
24. Mera SL, Lovell CR, Russell Jones R, Davies JD. Elastic fibers in normal and sun-damaged skin: an immunohistochemical study. *Br J Dermatol* 1987; 117: 21-7.
25. Davies JD, Young EW, Mera SL, Barnard K. Lysozyme is a component of human vascular elastic fibers. *Experimentia* 1983; 39: 382-3.
26. Park PW, Biedermann K, Mecham L, Bissett DL, Mecham RP. Lysozyme binds to elastin and protects elastin from elastase-mediated degradation. *J Invest Dermatol* 1996; 106: 1075-80.

Expression of DNA damage and stress proteins by UVA irradiation of human skin *in vivo*

Lee Ann Applegate, Corinne Scaletta, Anny Fourtanier, Romano E. Mascotto, Sophie Seité, Edgar Frenk

L.A. Applegate, C. Scaletta, E. Frenk: Department of Dermatology, Laboratory of Photobiology, University Hospital-CHUV BT-04-423, CH-1011 Lausanne, Switzerland.
A. Fourtanier, R.E. Mascotto, S. Seité: L'Oréal, Centre de Recherche Charles-Zviak, 90, rue du Général-Roguet, 92583 Clichy Cedex, France.

UV radiation of different wavelengths has been shown to alter proteins and induce nuclear factors in human cells *in vitro*. The *in vivo* effects on human skin and particularly those due to UVA are much less known. We therefore investigated in vivo the induction fo DNA damage and stress proteins by UVA I (340-450 nm, with small amount of visible) and UVA i + II (320-400 nm). Previously unexposed skin of 5 volunteers was irradiated with ~ 1 and 2 MED of UVA I and UVA I + II radiations, 4 mm biopsies were taken at 24 h post-UV and fresh frozen and formalin fixed, paraffin embedded 5 mm sections were prepared. Immunohistochemistry was performed with antibodies to ferritin, p53, NFkB and pyrimidine dimers. UVA I induced a dose-dependent marked expression of ferritin in suprabasal epidermal and interstitial dermal cells, which was not obtained by UVA I + II. Induction of p53 induction also varied occording to the UVA spectrum used : UVA I + II was more efficient and produced staining throughout the epidermis, whereas UVA I only induced detectable effects in basal cell of the epidermis. Pyrimidine dimer induction was marked following both UVA I and UVA I + II radiations: following UVA I, it could be detected well into the dermis. NFkB was induced in a dose-dependent manner following both radiations in epidermal keratinocytes. Our experiments have demonstrated that 1 to 2 MED of UVA radiation induce *in vivo* in human skin easily detectable alterations depending on the UVA spectrum used.

Human exposure to ultraviolet radiation from sunlight can cause many adverse effects including sunburn, premature aging, cataract formation, immune suppression and skin cancer [1-8]. The UVB region of the sun's spectrum (290-320 nm) was generally thought to be the most deleterious portion of sunlight. However, UVA radiation (320-400 nm) which penetrates deeply into skin is also potentially carcinogenic, can cause a wide variety of biological effects similar to those already seen induced by the UVB spectrum [3, 7-11] and was recently classified as a human carcinogen (International Agency for Research on Cancer, IARC). The cellular modifications induced by UVA radiation, unlike those produced by UVB, have considerable similarities to those induced by oxidative damages [12].

Studies on UVA radiation have taken a precedent in recent years. Some of the reasons for the increased interest in the UVA spectrum include: (1) photosensitivity reactions are mostly mediated by UVA; (2) UVA in conjunction with photosensitizing drugs has permitted vast therapeutic possibilities in chronic skin disorders; (3) high intensity sources of UVA are now widely used in tanning salons and for home usage; (4) the majority of sunscreens effectively block or diminish the UVB spectrum but this is not yet the case for the UVA spectrum. In Europe, the availability of high energy UVA sources is non-regulated. One can even find coin-operated tanning salons open 24 h a day and thus allowing a person to accumulate very high levels of radiation exposure. From a human health standpoint, it is important to know what effects are produced by these wavelengths.

Materials and methods

Radiation sources

A UVASUN 3000 lamp (Mutzhas, Munich, Germany) was used at a dose rate of 500-600 W/m^2 at a distance of 60-90 cm. Irradiation periods were within the range of 5-30 min. The spectral output of the lamp was analyzed with a calibrated Optronic model 742 spectroradiometer (Optronics Laboratories Inc., Orlando, FL, USA) and showed a broad peak between 360 and 410 nm *(Fig. 1)*. Before and after each experiment, radiation fluences were monitored by an International Light Radiometer (IL 1700, calibrated against the spectroradiometer). This radiation is termed UVA I even though there is a very small amount of visible light present.

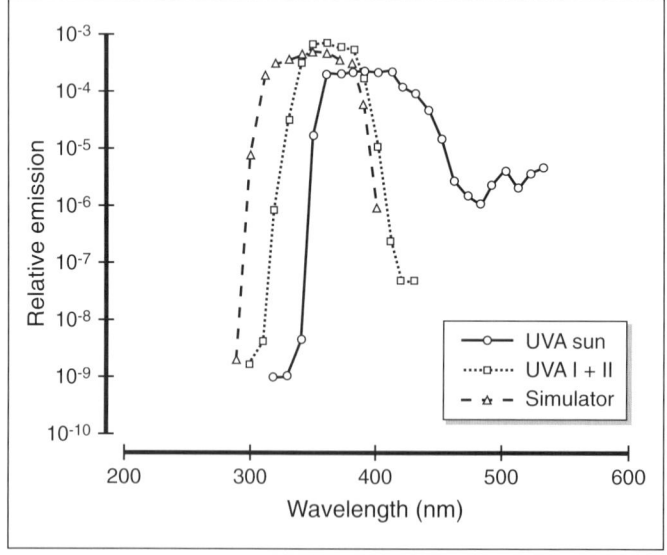

Figure 1. *Relative emission spectra of various lamps measured with a spectroradiometer at 10 nm intervals.*

An additional constructed filter, permitting combined UVA I and UVA II radiation without visible light (320-400 nm) was also adapted to the UVASUN 3000 lamp and used at a dose rate of 700-800 W/m^2 at a distance of 60-90 cm. Irradiation periods were within the range of 3-20 minutes. The spectral measurements were as described above. This radiation is termed UVA I + II *(Fig. 1)*.

A 15S single port Solar UV Simulator filtered with Schott WG320/1 mm and UG 11/1 mm filters (290-400 nm) emitting energy similar to that of the overhead sun up to 400 nm *(Fig. 1)* was used at a dose rate of 13-16 W/m^2 (Solar Light Company, Philadelphia, Penn. USA). Irradiation periods were approximately of 2 min duration. Radiation exposure (intensity and dose) were continuously controlled by a Dose Control System (Solar Light Company) directly attached to the 15S Solar Simulator which automatically operates a shutter system that closes for a preset dose.

Volunteers and irradiation *in vivo*

Healthy volunteers, between the ages of 20 and 60 with skin type I-IV, were used in these studies. Delimited areas of the buttocks were subjected to increasing doses of UVA I radiation (25, 50, 75 and 100 J/cm^2) and UVA I + II radiation (15, 35 and 70 J/cm^2). Biopsies of 4 mm were taken under local anesthesia (1% lidocaine) 30 min to 72 h following UVA radiation at ~1 and 2 minimal erythema doses (MED) and from an adjacent non-irradiated control site.

Some biopsies were immediately placed in a beaker with isopentane-2-methyl-butane chilled in liquid nitrogen for 2 min. Thereafter, the tissue was transferred to liquid nitrogen for storage until frozen serial sections of 5 µm could be prepared. Other biopsies were placed in formalin for fixation and blocked in paraffin for subsequent 5 µm serial sections.

Immunohistochemistry

Frozen sections of 5 µm thickness and fixed tissue were used for the immunohistochemistry. All incubations were done in a humidified chamber unless otherwise specified. Frozen sections were fixed with 4% paraformaldehyde for 30 min at 25° C and washed with PBS 3 times for 10 min each. Tissue sections were incubated with 0.1% phenylhydrazine in PBS for 60 min at 37° C to block endogenous peroxidases and washed twice for 5 min each. Nonspecific binding was blocked by an incubation for 2 h at 25° C with a solution of PBS containing 5% fetal calf serum (FCS), 7% normal goat serum (NGS), and 0.1% Triton X 100.

Tissue sections were then incubated overnight at 4° C with respective antibodies at various dilutions in PBS containing 5% FCS, 5% NGS and 0.1% Triton X 100 (ferritin, 1 : 20,000, Sigma; NFκB, 1 : 2,000, Serotec; p53, 1 : 200, Dako; thymine dimers, 1 : 300; H3 antibody provided by Dr. Len Rosa). The following morning, tissue sections were washed 3 times for 10 min each in PBS and were treated with biotinylated goat anti-rabbit at 1:200 in a solution of PBS with 5% FCS, 1% NGS, and 0.1% Triton X 100 for 3 h at 25° C. Tissue sections were washed 4 times for 5 min each in PBS and then treated with Vectastain ABC® (Vector, Burlingame, CA) as indicated by the company for 3 h at 25° C. After this incubation, tissue sections were washed 3 times for 10 min each in PBS and treated with 0.5 mg/ml 3,3'-diaminobenzidine with 0.32 µl 30% H$_2$O$_2$ added just before an incubation of 1-2 min. All samples were treated at the same time. The samples were washed for 5 min under running water. They were counterstained with Papanicolaou (Harris' hematoxylin solution), dehydrated and mounted with Merckoglas® (Merck).

Erythema measurements

Erythema measurements were taken immediately and 24 h following the UV exposure of skin. Measurements were taken for each individual by the same investigator with a DermaSpectrometer® (Cortex Technology, Denmark). This instrument calculates an erythema index by comparing the amount of non-specular, reflected red and green light relative to a white standard (where hemoglobin absorbs in the green interval, 520-580 nm with minimal absorption in the red, > 600 nm).

The results are thus presented as relative values of erythema which were an average of 3 measures. In all experiments, background measurements were taken from 2 regions parallel to the irradiated skin and were subtracted from the values obtained from irradiated areas.

Results

Erythema responses following UVA I and UVA II irradiation

Erythema responses varied considerably depending on which wavelengths were used and whether or not the skin site had been previously exposed to sunlight. Erythema induction could be produced easily and was reproducible to the same degree on non-exposed buttock skin with UVA I and UVA I + II regardless of skin type (skin types I-IV). The erythema produced by UVA I and UVA I + II was similar and appeared at approximately the same time as that routinely induced by UVB or solar simulating light on non-sun-exposed skin sites.

In contrast were the results obtained on previously exposed forearm skin using these same wavebands. UVA I did not produce a readily visible or reproducible erythema whereas irradiation with UVA I + II produced a measurable erythema when measured with a Dermaspectrometer® *(Fig. 2)*.

Induction of stress proteins in human skin *in vivo*

Cellular defense against UVA radiation seems to have more similarities with antioxidant pathways than it does with DNA repair pathways which are necessary to eliminate primarily induced DNA damage by UVC (190-290 nm) and UVB radiation [13].

Because the skin is in continual contact with the external environment, its' ability to provide protection against oxidative damage due to toxic chemicals and radiation is a primordial function. There exists a vast repertoire of antioxidant defenses in human skin cells including

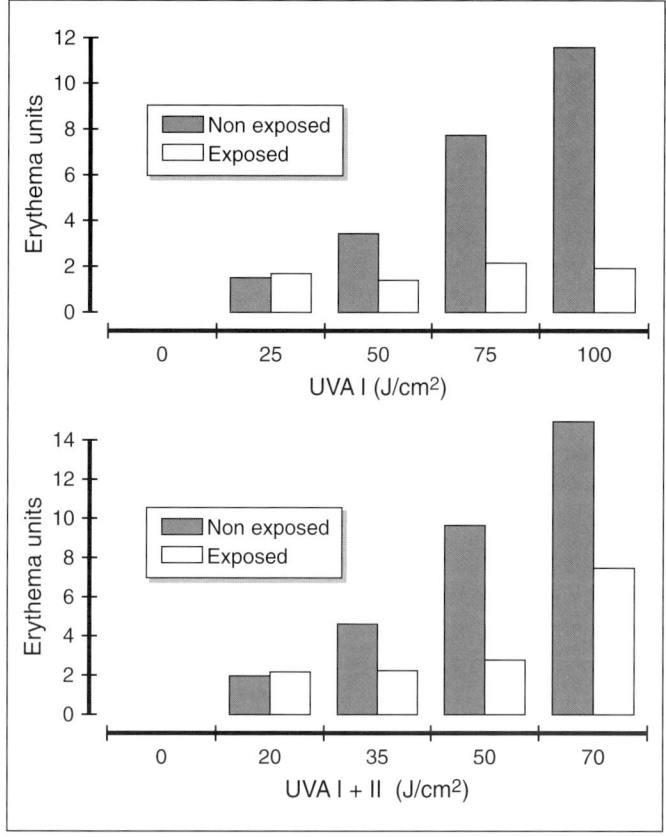

Figure 2. *Erythema dose responses measured on non-exposed and exposed sites from individuals with skin types 1-IV following UVA I and UVA I + II irradiation.*

antioxidant enzymes (*e.g.* superoxide dismutase, catalase, glutathione peroxidase, glutathione reductase) as well as lipophilic (tocopherol and ubiquinol) and hydrophilic (glutathione, ascorbate) antioxidants [14, 15]. In addition to the constitutive high level of the heme catabolizing enzyme, hemeoxygenase-2 (HO-2), there is also an inducible defense system in human skin fibroblasts which involves the isoform HO-1 [16-25]. The discovery that the HO-1 gene is strongly induced in cultured human skin fibroblasts by oxidants including UVA has provided the first example of a marked gene induction by an oxidizing carcinogen. Induction of HO-1 in fibroblasts was shown to correlate with an enhancement of cellular ferritin levels [21, 22].

Ferritin constitutes the major storage site for non-metabolized, intracellular iron and therefore plays a critical role in regulating the availability of iron to catalyze such harmful reactions as the peroxidation of lipids and the production of hydroxy radicals by the Fenton reaction. In cultured skin fibroblasts, it has been shown that the increase in ferritin levels constitutes an adaptive response that serves to protect these cells from subsequent oxidative membrane damage [21]. In cultured epidermal keratinocytes, ferritin levels are 3-7 fold higher than in dermal fibroblasts [24, 26] and it has been suggested that the observed high levels of ferritin are a constitutive response mediated by increased levels of antioxidants [21].

We attempted to identify where the putative protective protein, ferritin, resides in human skin and also whether or not it is perturbed following oxidative stress by UVA radiation.

Ferritin staining of normal human skin from previously non-exposed body sites (buttocks) was readily detected in both epidermal and dermal tissue along with associated structures (*i.e.* hair follicles, vessel walls, muscles, sebaceous glands). Most remarkable was the specific staining of the basal keratinocyte layer of the epidermis where some heterogeneity in staining intensity was seen among the five individuals tested. Basal keratinocytes of hair follicles were also moderately stained. Within the papillary dermis, isolated cells, most likely dermal fibroblasts, were weak to moderately stained depending on the individual. Within the reticular dermis these cells were weakly stained. Vessel walls, muscles and sebaceous glands also showed weak ferritin staining.

Immunohistochemical analysis of biopsies from sites irradiated with dose of 0, 50 and 100 J/cm^2 of UVA I show a definite increase in epidermal ferritin staining at 24 h post-UVA. The suprabasal layer and isolated spinous keratinocytes became stained following these doses of UVA radiation. Suprabasal keratinocytes of hair follicles also had increased staining for ferritin following these doses of UVA I. In both the papillary and reticular dermis, ferritin stained cells were shown to increase subtantially following UVA I radiation in a dose dependent manner. No changes in ferritin staining were seen in vessel walls, muscles or sebaceous glands.

Following UVA I + II irradiation of the buttocks of the same volunteers, no remarkable changes were noted in the epidermis following 35 and 70 J/cm^2 at 24 h.

Alterations in the dermis were similar to those seen with UVA I (with slightly lower prevalence), with numbers of interstitial and perivascular cells showing increased staining.

Alteration of NFκB in human skin *in vivo*

Nuclear factor κB is a transcription factor that has been reported to be activated *in vitro* by ultraviolet radiation and recently by UVA I [27]. NFκB responsive elements are required for the functioning of many cytokine promoters and play a central role in the induction of many immunoregulatory genes. *In vivo*, rare staining of NFκB was seen in normal non-irradiated buttock skin in the epidermal layers. Following 50 and 100 J/cm^2 of UVA I, there was an increased staining of NFκB throughout the upper layers of the epidermis. A similar effect was seen with UVA I + II radiation with staining apparent throughout the epidermis and with slightly more basal cell layer involvement than that seen with UVA I.

Induction of DNA damage and p53 in human skin *in vivo*

Ultraviolet radiation induces DNA damage which has been shown to be responsible for a variety of negative effects in human skin. More recently, skin appears to respond to DNA damage with positive actions. Skin appears to possess a p53-dependent "guardian of the tissue" response to DNA damage in a pathway which aborts precancerous cells [28]. It has previously been shown that UV radiation can induce p53 *in vivo* [29] and we wanted to look at the distribution of induction of pyrimidine dimers and p53 following both UVA I and UVA I + II irradiation in previously non-sun-exposed human skin.

Pyrimidine dimers induced by ultraviolet radiation have been shown to be responsible for many biological effects in skin including erythema, sunburn cell formation, suppressed immunity of the skin and tumor formation [1-4].

These lesions could be readily detected following 50 and 100 J/cm^2 UVA I radiation with staining seen well into the papillary and reticular dermis using the H3 antibodies which detect thymine dimers (Dr Len Rosa). High epidermal staining with relatively little staining of the papillary dermis was also seen following UVA I + II irradiation of the buttock skin of the same individuals *(Fig. 3)*. Interestingly, control biopsies taken at various distances from the irradiated sites showed staining for dimers.

When biopsies were taken at 1 to 10 cm for irradiated skin with 50-100 J/cm^2, dimers could be detected easily at 2-3 cm from the original irradiation site but no longer at 10 cm. No increased staining was seen for ferritin, NFκB or p53 in the same biopsies. Induction of p53 was seen in the epidermis of previously non-exposed skin following 50 and 100 J/cm^2 of UVA I. A predominance of staining of basal cells of the epidermis was seen. Staining for p53 following UVA I + II at 24 h showed an involvement of all layers of the epidermis *(Fig. 3)*. Differences of these staining patterns for the UVA I and the UVA I + II spectra could be due to penetration properties or some aspect of basal cells in the epidermis.

Discussion

We have established that both UVA I and UVA I + II radiation can indeed induce stress proteins and DNA damage in human skin *in vivo* following acute sub-erythemal doses. The distribution of staining throughout the epidermis and dermis depends greatly on the wavelengths as only small shifts in the spectrum can show significant differences.

Although it is essential to study DNA damage and defense mechanisms on isolated cells in culture, it is also of importance to characterize these defined mechanisms at the tissue level where cell-cell interactions occur concomitantly. In this respect, we have seen that in skin, ferritin is globally induced following high doses of UVA radiation *in situ*. An increase in quantity of this antioxidant following UVA radiation could establish an environment of higher protection for further oxidative stress. Furthermore, ferritin expression could be used as an *in vivo* marker of UVA radiation-induced oxidative stress and thereby permit evaluation of the efficacy of applied UVA sunscreens. Likewise, the nuclear alterations induced by UVA radiation studied herein provide interesting, additional *in vivo* markers for such purposes.

Acknowledgements

The authors wish to thank the medical staff of the Dermatology Department (CHUV) for the biopsies of the volunteers and Dr. Len Rosa for the H3 antibodies. This study was supported in part by grants from the Swiss National Fund (LAA, EF 312-41846.94), the Stiftung für Krebs-bekämpfung, Zürich (EF and LAA), and by L'Oréal.

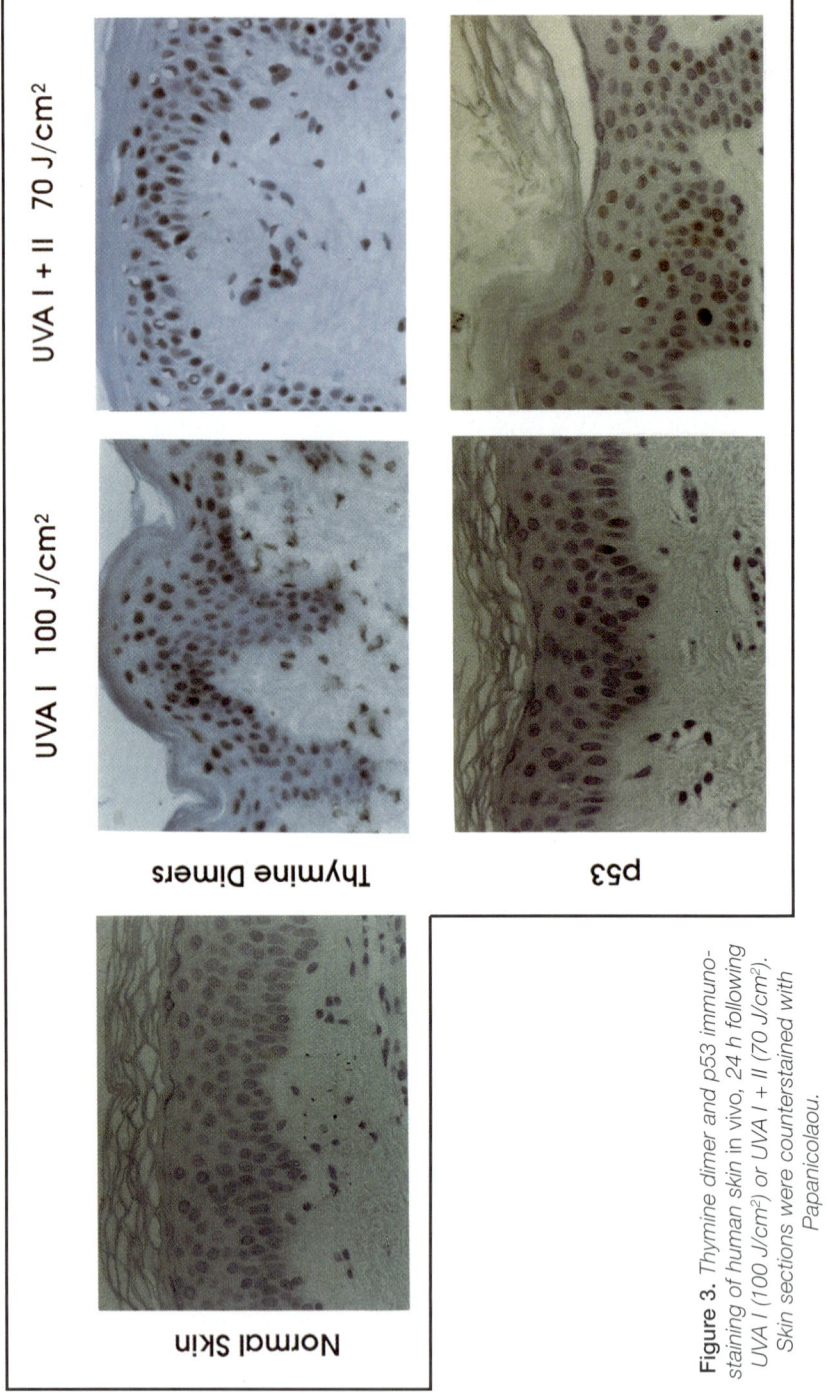

Figure 3. Thymine dimer and p53 immuno-staining of human skin in vivo, 24 h following UVA I (100 J/cm²) or UVA I + II (70 J/cm²). Skin sections were counterstained with Papanicolaou.

References

1. Jagger J. Multicellular Systems. In: Jagger J, ed. *Solar-UV actions on living cells*. New York: Praeger Press, 1985: 113-35.
2. Kripke ML, Applegate LA. Alteration in the immune response by ultraviolet radiation. In: Goldsmith LA, ed. *Biochemistry and physiology of the skin*. New York: Oxford Press, 2nd edition, 1991: 1304-28.
3. Parrish JA, Anderson RR, Urbach F, Pitts D. *UVA: biological effects of ultraviolet radiation with emphasis on human responses to longwave ultraviolet*. New York: Plenum Press, 1978.
4. Kripke ML. Immunologic mechanisms in UV radiation carcinogenesis. *Adv Cancer Res* 1981; 34: 69-106.
5. Applegate LA, Lautier D, Frenk E, Tyrrell RM. Endogenous glutathione levels modulate the frequency of both spontaneous and long wavelength ultraviolet induced mutations in human cells. *Carcinogenesis* 1992; 13: 1557-60.
6. Soter NA. Acute effects of ultraviolet radiation on the skin. Sem Dermatol 1990; 9: 11-5.
7. Gilchrest BA, Soter NA, Hawk JLM, Barr RM, Black AK, Hensby CN, Mallet AI, Greaves MW, Parrish JA. Histologic changes associated with ultraviolet A-induced erythema in normal human skin. *J Am Acad Dermatol* 1983; 9: 213-9.
8. Van Wheelden H, de Gruijl FR, van der Leun JC. Carcinogenesis by UVA, with an attempt to assess the carcinogenic risks of tanning with UVA and UVB. In: Urbach F, Gange RW, eds. *The biological effects of UVA radiation*. New York: Praeger Press, 1986: 137-46.
9. Morrey JD, Bourn SM, Bunch TD, Jackson MK, Sidwell RW, Barrows LR, Daynes RA, Rosen CA. In vivo activation of human immunodeficiency virus type 1 long terminal repeat by UV type A (UVA) light plus psoralen and UVB light in the skin of transgenic mice. *J Virology* 1991; 65: 5045-51.
10. Freeman SE, Gange RW, Matzinger EA, Sutherland JC, Sutherland BM. Production of pyrimidine dimers in human skin exposed *in situ* to UVA radiation. *J Invest Dermatol* 1987; 88: 430-3.
11. Rosario R, Mark GJ, Parrish JA. Histological changes produced in skin by equally erythemogenic doses of UVA, UVB, UVC and UVA with psoralens. *Br J Dermatol* 1979; 101: 299-308.
12. Tyrrell RM. UVA (320-380 nm) radiation as an oxidative stress. In: Sies H, ed. *Oxidative stress: oxidants and antioxidants*. New York: Academic Press, 1991: 57-78.
13. Applegate LA, Frenk E. Cellular defense mechanisms of the skin against oxidant stress and in particular UVA radiation. Eur J Dermatol 1995; 5: 97-103.
14. Yohn JJ, Norris DA, Yrastorza DG, Buno IJ, Leff JA, Hake SS. Disparate antioxidant enzyme activities in cultured human cutaneous fibroblasts, keratinocytes, and melanocytes. J Invest Dermatol 1991; 97: 405-9.
15. Shindo Y, Witt E, Han D, Epstein W, Packer L. Enzymatic and non-enzymatic antioxidants in epidermis and dermis of human skin. J Invest Dermatol 1994; 102: 122-4.
16. Keyse SM, Tyrrell RM. Both near and ultraviolet radiation and the oxidizing agent hydrogen peroxide induce the 32 kDa stress protein in normal human skin fibroblasts. *J Biol Chem* 1987; 262: 14821-5.
17. Keyse SM, Tyrrell RM. Heme oxygenase is the major 32 kDa stress protein induced in human skin fibroblasts by UVA radiation, hydrogen peroxide, and sodium arsenite. *Proc Natl Acad Sci USA* 1989; 86: 99-103.
18. Stocker R. Induction of haem oxygenase as a defence against oxidative stress. *Free Rad Res Comms* 1990; 9: 101-12.
19. Applegate LA, Luscher P, Tyrrell RM. Induction of heme oxygenase: a general response to oxidant stress in cultured mammalian cells. *Cancer Res* 1991; 51: 974-8.
20. Maines MD, Trakshel GM, Kutty RK. Characterization of two constitutive forms of rat liver microsomal heme oxygenase. Only one molecular species of the enzyme is inducible. *J Biol Chem* 1986; 261: 411-9.
21. Vile GF, Tyrrell RM. Oxidative stress resulting from ultraviolet A irradiation of human skin fibroblasts leads to a heme oxygenase-dependent increase in ferritin. *J Biol Chem* 1993; 268: 14678-81.

22. Vile GF, Basu-Modak S, Waltner C, Tyrrell RM. Haem oxygenase-1 mediates an adaptive response to oxidative stress in human skin fibroblasts. *Proc Natl Acad Sci USA* 1994; 91: 2607-10.
23. Balla G, Jacob HS, Rosenberg M, Nath K, Apple F, Eaton JW, Vercelloti GM. Ferritin: a cytoprotective antioxidant strategem of endothelium. *J Biol Chem* 1992; 267: 18148-53.
24. Applegate LA, Noel A, Vile G, Frenk E, Tyrrell RM. Two genes contribute to different extents to the heme oxygenase enzyme activity measured in cultured human skin fibroblasts and keratinocytes: implications for protection against oxidant stress. *Photochem Photobiol* 1995; 61: 285-91.
25. Lautier D, Luscher P, Tyrrell RM. Endogenous glutathione levels modulate both constitutive and UVA radiation/hydrogen peroxide inducible expression of the human heme oxygenase gene. *Carcinogen* 1992; 13: 227-32.
26. Applegate LA, Frenk E. Oxidative defence in cultured human skin fibroblasts and keratinocytes from sun-exposed and non-exposed skin. *Photoderm Photoimmunol Photmed* 1995; 11: 95-101.
27. Vile GF, Tanew-Liitschew A, Tyrrell RM. Activation of NFkB in human skin fibroblasts by the oxidative stress generated by UVA radiation. *Photochem Photobiol* 1995; 62: 463-8.
28. Hall PA, McKee PH, du P. Menage H, Dover R, Lane DP. High levels of p53 protein in UV-irradiated normal human skin. *Oncogene* 1993; 8: 203-7.
29. Ziegler A, Jonason AS, Leffell DJ, Simon JA, Sharma HW, Kimmelman J, Remington L, Jacks T, Brash DE. Sunburn and p53 in the onset of skin cancer. *Nature* 1994; 372: 773-6.

Mechanisms of UV-induced immunosuppression

Link between UV-induced tolerance and apoptosis

Thomas Schwarz

T. Schwarz: Department of Dermatology, University Münster, D-48149 Münster, Germany.

Exposure to UV light impairs sensitization to haptens applied directly to the irradiated skin area [1, 2]. In addition, hapten-specific tolerance develops, which is due to the generation of hapten-specific T suppressor cells [3]. Although the transfer of tolerance by injecting T cells from UV-exposed mice into naive recipients was described more than 10 years ago, the mechanisms by which T suppressor cells mediate tolerance still remain to be determined. There is increasing evidence that apoptosis plays an important role in immune reactions [4]. CD95, also called Fas or APO-1, is a surface molecule [5, 6] which induces apoptotic cell death following interaction with its natural CD95L, also called FasL [7]. Grafts of testis, a tissue which expresses high levels of FasL, surprisingly survive indefinitely when transplanted into allogeneic animals [8]. In contrast, when testis derived from *gld* mice which, due to a natural mutation lack functional FasL, are transplanted into allogeneic recipients, rejection occurs. This implies that testis cells, *via* expression of FasL, kill attacking T cells of the host and thereby escape the immune response. Similar mechanisms have been observed for a variety of tumor cells, explaining the immune privileged status of these cells [9].

Since tolerance can be considered as a form of immune privilege, we became interested as to whether the Fas/FasL system is important for UV-induced tolerance. To address this issue we utilized *lpr* mice which lack functional Fas and *gld* mice which lack functional FasL [10, 11]. Exposure of both strains to low doses of UV light inhibited the induction of contact hypersensitivity following application of the hapten DNFB to UV-irradiated skin. Since in this respect *lpr* and *gld* mice behaved in a similar way to C3H/HeN wild type mice, this suggests that *lpr* and *gld* mice with C3H/HeN background are UV-susceptible. In contrast to UV-exposed C3H mice, UV-exposed *lpr* and *gld* mice did not develop tolerance, because both strains revealed a significant contact hypersensitivity response upon resensitization about 3 weeks after UV-exposure. This clearly suggested that the Fas/FasL system is crucial for the development of tolerance [12]. These findings were confirmed by adoptive transfer experiments which showed that UV-mediated suppression is not transferable either in *lpr* or *gld* mice. Since *lpr* and *gld* mice were of the same genetic background (C3H/HeN), cross transfer experiments could be performed to clarify whether for the transfer of tolerance Fas and FasL, respectively, need to be expressed in the donor or in the recipient. Suppression was observed not only when cells from UV-exposed and hapten-treated *lpr* donors were injected into naive C3H mice, but also when cells from UV-exposed and hapten-treated *gld* mice were transferred into naive C3H mice. In contrast, both naive *lpr* and naive *gld* recipients of T suppressor cells from UV-exposed and hapten-treated C3H mice could be normally sensitized. Thus, these findings suggested that the transfer of tolerance does not require Fas or FasL expression on the suppressor cells but requires both molecules on cells in the recipient [12].

These findings were compatible with the hypothesis that T suppressor cells do not kill their targets *via* expression of CD95L themselves, but rather drive cells in the recipient that are essential during sensitization, into apoptosis and that this may be mediated *via* the Fas/FasL system. To test whether antigen-presenting cells undergo apoptosis when presenting the hapten in the presence of T suppressor cells, coincubation experiments with bone marrow-derived dendritic cells and T cells obtained from naive, sensitized or UV-tolerized (*i.e.* animals which were sensitized through UV-exposed skin) mice were performed. Death of dendritic cells was evaluated by FACS analysis (propidium iodide incorporation). Upon coincubation with T cells from sensitized mice in the presence of hapten around one third of the dendritic cells died which may be explained by activation-induced cell death. However, when dendritic cells were coincubated with T cells obtained from UV-tolerized mice, a significantly increased death rate of dendritic cells was detected [12]. This implies that T suppressors may mediate their inhibitory property by inducing apoptosis of antigen-presenting cells. The Fas/FasL system appears to be crucially involved since dendritic cells obtained from either *lpr* or *gld* mice were resistant to T suppressor cell-induced death. Together, these data suggest that T suppressor cells appear to exert their inhibitory capacity by inducing death of antigen-presenting cells which carry the specific hapten, and that cell death might be mediated *via* the Fas/FasL system.

Recently, we and others reported that interleukin-12 (IL-12) can break established UV-induced tolerance [13-15], the underlying mechanism, however, still remains unclear [16]. Interestingly, addition of IL-12 to cocultures of T suppressor cells and dendritic cells significantly reduced the number of dead dendritic cells [12]. This suggests that IL-12 may break tolerance by preventing dendritic cells from undergoing cell death induced by T suppressor cells. Since Fas/FasL expression appears essential, we presently speculate that IL-12 may influence the expression of CD95 and/or CD95L on dendritic cells.

Taken together, these data provide strong evidence for an important link between the apoptosis-associated Fas/FasL system and immune tolerance by demonstrating that the Fas/FasL system is essentially involved in mediating UV-induced tolerance. The data further indicate that T suppressor cells may induce cell death of antigen-presenting cells in the presence of the specific hapten, and that the Fas/FasL system is crucially involved in this process. IL-12 appears to rescue antigen-presenting cells from suppressor cell-induced cell death, a mechanism which may be responsible for its ability to break established tolerance.

References

1. Toews GB, Bergstresser PR, Streilein JW. Epidermal Langerhans cell density determines whether contact hypersensitivity or unresponsiveness follows skin painting with DNFB. *J Immunol* 1980; 124: 445-53.
2. Cooper KD, Oberhelman L, Hamilton TA, Baadsgaard O, Terhune M, Le Vee G, Anderson T, Koren H. UV exposure reduces immunization rates and promotes tolerance to epicutaneous antigens in humans: relationship to dose $CD1a^-DR^+$ epidermal macrophage induction, and Langerhans cell depletion. *Proc Natl Acad Sci USA* 1992; 89: 8497-501.
3. Elmets CA, Bergstresser PR, Tigelaar RE, Wood PJ, Streilein JW. Analysis of the mechanism of unresponsiveness produced by haptens painted on skin exposed to low dose ultraviolet radiation. *J Exp Med* 1983; 158: 781-94.
4. Lynch DH, Ramsdell F, Alderson MR. Fas and FasL in the homeostatic regulation of immune responses. *Immunol Today* 1995; 16: 569-74.

5. Itoh M, Yonehara S, Ishii A, Yonehara M, Mizushima SI, Sameshima M, Hase A, Seta Y, Nagata S. The polypeptide encoded by the cDNA for human cell surface antigen Fas can mediate apoptosis. *Cell* 1991; 66: 233-43.
6. Trauth BC, Klas C, Peters AMJ, Matzku S, Moller P, Falk W, Debatin KM, Krammer PH. Monoclonal antibody-mediated tumor regression by induction of apoptosis. *Science* 1998; 245: 301-5.
7. Suda T, Takahashi T, Golstein P, Nagata S. Molecular cloning and expression of the Fas ligand, a novel member of the tumor necrosis factor family. *Cell* 1993; 75: 1169-78.
8. Bellgrau D, Gold D, Selawry H, Moore J, Franzusoff A, Duke RC. A role for Fas ligand in preventing graft rejection. *Nature* 1995; 377: 630-2.
9. Hahne M, Rimoldi D, Schröter M, Romero P, Schreier M, French LE, Schneider P, Bornaand T, Fontana A, Lienard D, Cerottini JC, Tshopp J. Melanoma cell expression of Fas (APO-1/CD95) ligand: implications for tumor immune escape. *Science* 1996; 274-1363-6.
10. Watanabe-Fukunaga R, Brannan CI, Copeland NG, Jenkins NA, Nagata S. Lymphoproliferation disorder in mice explained by defects in Fas antigen that mediates apoptosis. *Nature* 1992; 356: 314-7.
11. Takahashi T, Tanaka M, Brannan CA, Jenkins NA, Copeland NG, Suda T, Nagata S. Generalized lymphoproliferative disease in mice caused by a point mutation in the Fas ligand. *Cell* 1994; 76: 969-76.
12. Schwars A, Grabbe S, Grosse-Heitmeyer K, Roters B, Riemann H, Luger TA, Trinchieri G, Schwarz T. Ultraviolet light induced immune tolerance is mediated via the CD95/CD95-ligand system. *J Immunol* 1998 (in press).
13. Schmitt DA, Owen-Schaub L, Ullrich SE. Effect of IL-12 on immune suppression and suppressor cell induction by ultraviolet radiation. *J Immunol* 1995; 154: 5114-20.
14. Müller G, Saloga J, Germann T, Schuler G, Knop J, Enk AH. IL-12 as mediator and adjuvant for the induction of contact sensitivity *in vivo*. *J Immunol* 1995; 155: 4661-8.
15. Schwarz A, Grabbe S, Aragane Y, Sandkuhl K, Riemann H, Luger TA, Kubin M, Trinchieri G, Schwarz T. Interleukin-12 prevents UVB-induced local immunosuppression and overcomes UVB-induced tolerance. *J Invest Dermatol* 1996; 106: 1187-91.
16. Schwarz A, Grabbe S, Mahnke K, Riemann H, Luger TA, Wysocka M, Trinchieri G, Schwarz T. IL-12 breaks UV light induced immunosuppression by affecting CD8+ rather than CD4+ T cells. *J Invest Dermatol* 1988 (in press).

Dose-responses for UV-induced suppression of various immune responses

Taihong Kim, Stephen E. Ullrich, Margaret L. Kripke

T. Kim, S.E. Ullrich, M.L. Kripke: Department of Immunology, The University of Texas, M.D. Anderson Cancer Center, Houston, TX, USA.

Many immunological assays have been used to measure UV-induced immune suppression, including tumor rejection, contact and delayed hypersensitivity responses, antibody production, and number and function of epidermal Langerhans cells. Whether all of these assays depend on the same UV-initiated sequence of events is not clear; therefore, careful studies of the UV dose-responses and wavelength dependencies might be useful in indicating differences and similarities in the mechanisms by which UV suppresses various immune reactions. In addition, such information is critical for assessing the ability of sunscreens to protect against UV-induced immune suppression. We therefore carried out a series of UV dose-response studies for suppression of various immunologic responses in C3H mice after a single exposure to FS40 sunlamps, kodacel-filtered FS40 sunlamps, or a solar UV simulator. The assays included local and systemic suppression of contact hypersensitivity (CHS) to DNFB and systemic suppression of delayed-type hypersensitivity (DTH) to *Candida albicans* and alloantigen. The mice were immunized 3 days after UV at the site of irradiation (local suppression) or at a distant site (systemic suppression).

With all assays, the FS40 sunlamp was the most efficient in inducing immune suppression, followed by the kodacel-filtered FS40, followed by the solar simulator. This is not unexpected since shorter wavelengths of UV-B are known to be more efficient in suppressing CHS responses than longer UV-B or UV-A wavelengths, and FS40 lamps have the greatest amount of short UV-B and the solar simulator, the least. Comparison of the dose responses for suppression of the 4 immune responses using a single UV source showed that the UV-B dose required to achieve 50% suppression was least for local suppression of CHS to DNFB, followed by systemic suppression of DTH to *C. albicans*, CHS to DNFB, and DTH to alloantigen. This order was the same with all 3 UV sources. Calculated regression lines for suppression of the 4 assays were not parallel. From this study, we concluded that the dose-responses for suppression of a given inmune response differ with different UV spectra and that the UV dose-responses for suppression of an immune response differ depending on the assay (DTH *vs* CHS), the site of antigen administration (irradiated *vs* non-irradiated), and the antigen itself (DTH to *C. albicans vs* alloantigen).

We next investigated the initiating event in photosuppression of the two DTH responses using antibody against cis-urocanic acid (UCA) or liposomes containing T4 endonuclease V (T4N5 liposomes). Suppression of DTH to *C. albicans* was completely reversed by applying T4N5 liposomes to the skin immediately after irradiation, but was unaffected by injection of anti-cis-UCA antibody. Conversely, suppression of DTH to alloantigen was unaffected by T4N5 liposome application, but was restored by anti-cis-UCA antibody. We conclude that different mechanisms are involved in suppression of the DTH response to different antigens by UV radiation and speculate that this may be due to differences in the particular antigen-presenting cell population utilized by a particular antigen. These findings imply that a single immunological assay may be insufficient to measure photoprotection against UV-induced immune suppression.

UV-induced immunosuppression.
The critical role of wavelength

Bert Jan Vermeer, M. Wintzen, F.H.J. Claas, A.A. Schothorst, H.M.H. Hurks

Bert Jan Vermeer, M. Wintzen, A.A. Schothorst, H.M.H. Hurks: Department of Dermatology, University Hospital Leiden, P.O. Box 9600, 2300 RC. Leiden, The Netherlands.
F.H.J. Claas: Immunohematology and Blood Bank, University Medical Center Leiden, Leiden, The Netherlands.

Ultraviolet radiation has been shown to modify cutaneous immune responses, a phenomenon that is called photo-immunosuppression [1, 2]. The mixed lymphocyte reaction (MLR) and mixed epidermal cell lymphocyte reaction (MECLR) are commonly used methods to study the effects of UVB radiation. These studies show that the alloactivating capacity of cells is decreased by UVB exposure. However, the mechanisms by which the suppression is achieved is still a matter of debate. Many *in vitro* and *in vivo* experiments in different species (rats, mice, humans) have been performed, often lead to contradictory results. We investigated the importance of irradiance and wavelength in the UV-induced suppression of the MLR and MECLR.

The influence of irradiance on the MECLR was studied *in vitro* using two Philips FS40 lamps, which have a major peak at 312 nm and 65% of the total energy within the UVB range (280-320 nm). The irradiance can be varied without changing the wavelength spectrum. Epidermal stimulator cells were exposed to UVB and cultured with responder PBMC in the MECLR for 6 days. Several doses of (total) UV were tested (10 80 mJ/cm^2) using two intensities of UV radiation (2.4 W/m^2 and 7.0 W/m^2). Irradiation of epidermal cells with high irradiance impaired the alloactivating capacity more than irradiation with low irradiance [3].

To obtain a better understanding of the mechanism by which UVB radiation decreases the allostimulating capacity of *in vitro* irradiated cells, we determined UV action spectra for both the MLR and MECLR. Suspensions of PBMC or epidermal cells were irradiated with monochromatic UV and used as stimulator cells in the MLR or MECLR. For irradiations at wavelengths of 254, 297 and 302 nm, a 1,000 W mercury-xenon arc lamp with interference filters of 254, 297 or 302 nm ± 4.0 half bandwidth (Oriel Corp., Stamford, CT) was used. Irradiation at 312 nm was performed with a bank of three 40 W TL-01 lamps (Philips), emitting the majority of their radiant energy (51%) at a peak at 312 nm. At all wavelengths, the MLR and MECLR responses decreased in a dose-dependent manner. In the MLR less UV light was needed to abrogate the alloactivating capacity of the irradiated cells. For determination of the action spectra, the slope of each individual dose-response curve was calculated. The fluence unit was converted from J/m^2 to photons/m^2. The mean slopes at each wavelength were normalized to 1.0 at 254 nm for plotting the action spectra. Both MLR and MECLR action spectra had a maximum at 254 nm and a relative sensitivity at 312 nm that was a thousand times lower than at 254 nm [4]. Strikingly, the action spectra corresponded very closely to the action spectra that were found [5] for the induction of thymine dimers and (6-4) photoproducts in irradiated calf thymus DNA solutions *(Fig. 1)*. This suggests strongly that the UV-induced abrogation of the MLR and MECLR responses is mediated by UV-induced DNA damage. Furthermore, the action spectra for the MLR and MECLR were similar, suggesting that they share a common mechanism for UV-induced suppression.

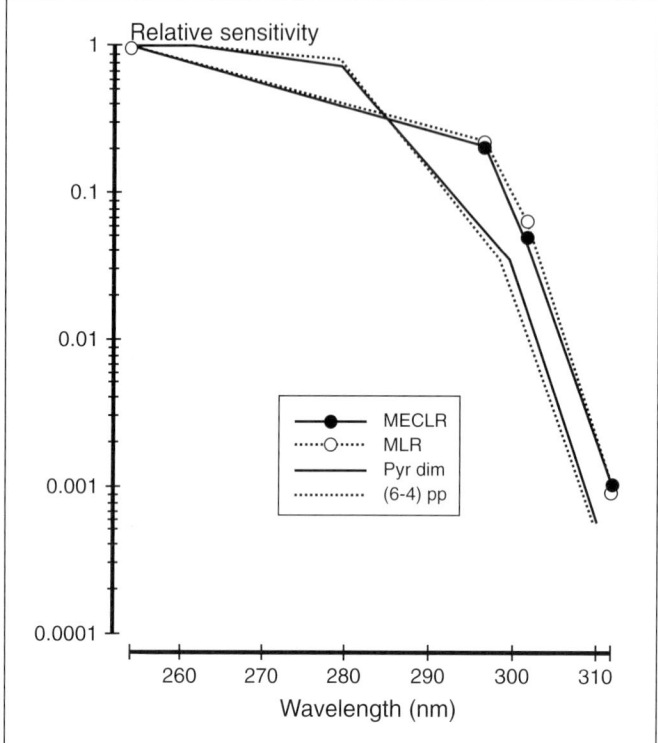

Figure 1. Action spectra for the MLR, MECLR, formation of pyrimidine dimers and formation of (6-4) photoproducts in the UV region from 254 nm to 312 nm (from Photochem Photobiol 1995; 62: 451).

All experiments described so far are *in vitro* studies. An *in vivo* spectrum for the induction of photo-immunosuppression in humans is not yet published. However, an action spectrum for the UV-induced suppression of contact hypersensitivity in mice has been published by De Fabo and Noonan [6]. This action spectrum corresponded with the DNA action spectrum only for wavelengths less than 290 nm. On the other hand, the action spectrum was very similar to the absorption spectrum of urocanic acid (UCA). Trans-UCA is a component of the stratum corneum and is isomerized to *cis*-UCA by UV radiation. It was suggested that *cis*-UCA plays an important role in photo-immunosuppression. Gibbs *et al.* [7] and Kammeyer *et al.* [8] have shown in mice and in humans and *in vitro* as well as *in vivo*, that next to UVB, UVA can also efficiently isomerize *trans*-UCA. These data might suggest that UV-induced immunosuppression *in vivo* is primarily mediated by DNA damage for wavelengths less than 290 nm and mediated by *cis*-UCA at higher wavelengths into the UVA region. Interestingly, Gibbs *et al.* [7] noted that UVA was capable of inducing *cis*-UCA whilst failing to suppress contact hypersensitivity, making the relationship between *cis*-UCA formation in skin and UV-induced immunosuppression complex.

We studied the effect of *cis*-UCA on the human MLR and MECLR *in vitro*. Addition of *cis*-UCA (6-100 µg) resulted in a 20% suppression of the MECLR, but not the MLR. Addition of *trans*-UCA did not affect the MECLR and MLR. *Cis*-UCA was not able to potentiate a sub-optimal UVB- or histamine-induced suppression of the MECLR. Although *in vivo cis*-UCA can mimic the effects of UVB radiation, *in vitro* we could only obtain a moderate suppression of the MECLR. This suggests again that the mode of action of *cis*-UCA must be complex, probably in cooperation with other immune mediators (*e.g.* IL-10, TNFα, PGE$_2$) and thus very difficult to mimic in an *in vitro* system. These studies show that UV-induced immunosuppression is dependent on the wavelength spectrum and on the irradiance of the UV source. Suppression of the MLR and MECLR by UV radiation *in vitro* is mediated by UV-induced DNA damage. *In vivo*, both DNA damage and UCA may play a role, possibly DNA damage more in the low-UVB region and UCA more in the UVA region.

One of the new candidates which may play a role in photo-immunosuppression are neuropeptides [9]. In preliminary data we could observe that exposure of cultured keratinocytes to physiological doses of UVA (Sellas lamp, 340-400 nm) caused a release of propiomelanocortin-related peptides [10, 11]. These peptides may have an effect on the immune system. The UVA irradiation may even cause the excretion of β endorphins from keratinocytes and may lead to an increased level of β-endorphins in the circulation. Therefore, this release of β-endorphins can have an effect on the feeling of wellbeing of the individual who receives UVA irradiation.

Ultraviolet irradiation may cause cellular damage and result in the inhibition of the proliferation potential of the irradiated cells. The keratinocytes and melanocytes are the cellular targets which are predominantly exposed to UV irradiation. For this reason we determined the UV-action spectra for survival of the keratinocytes and melanocytes. The cultured cells were irradiated with a mercury-xenon arc lamp equipped with narrow band interference filters as described earlier. The following wavelength were investigated (254, 297, 302, 365 nm). For irradiation with 312 nm three 40W Philips T1-01 lamps were used, which emit the majority (*i.e.* 51%) of their radiant energy at about 312 nm wavelength. After irradiation the cells were plated and colony formation was determined. As shown in *Figure 2* the inhibition of colony formation was primarily observed within the UVB range. The keratinocytes and melanocytes had

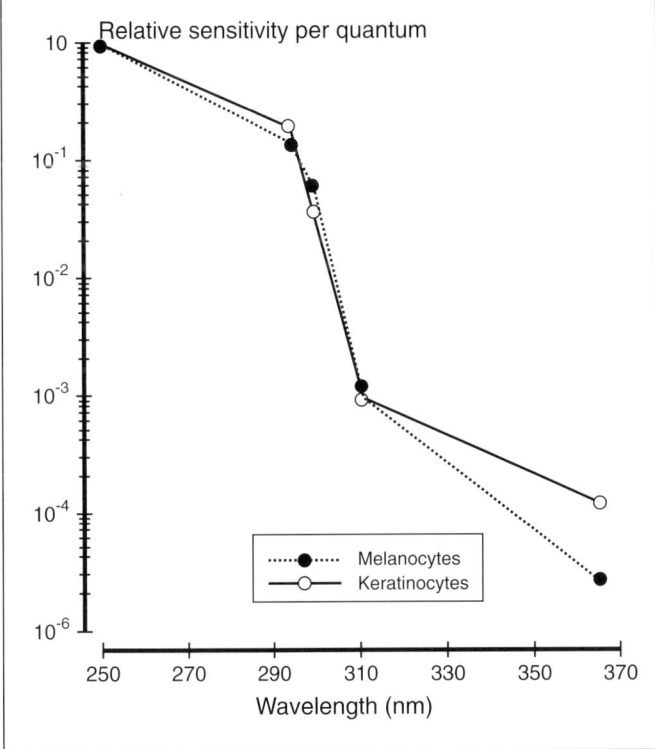

Figure 2. *Relative action spectra for cell survival (the reciprocal of D10) after quantum correction. The normalization was related to 254 nm light (from Photochem Photobiol 1994; 59: 433).*

the same sensitivity for UVB irradiation in our model. However when the cells were irradiated with UVA (wavelength 365 nm) the melanocytes were relatively less sensitive to UVA induced damage [12]. From these investigations we conclude that UVA might cause the following effects: (1) a slight inhibition of the immune response as measured by MLR and MECLR; (2) induction of the secretion of propiomelanocortin-related peptides by keratinocytes; (3) inhibition of the growth potential of keratinocytes and melanocytes (UVA is less cytotoxic to melanocytes than to keratinocytes).

References

1. Kripke ML. Immunological unresponsiveness induced by ultraviolet radiation. *Immunol Rev* 1984; 90: 87-107.
2. Vermeer BJ, Hurks MHM. The clinical relevance of immunosuppression by UV irradiation. *J Photochem Photobiol* 1994; 24: 149-54.
3. Hurks MHM, Out-Luiting C, Vermeer BJ, Claas FHJ, Mommaas AM. UVB-induced suppression of the mixed epidermal cell lymphocyte reaction is critically dependent on irradiance. *Photochem Photobiol* 1995; 62: 485-9.
4. Hurks MHM, Out-Luiting C, Vemeer BJ, Claas FHJ, Mommaas AM. The action spectra for UV-induced suppression of MLR and MECLR show that immunosuppression is mediated by DNA damage. *Photochem Photobiol* 1995; 62: 449-53.
5. Matsunaga T, Hieda K, Nikaido O. Wavelength dependent formation of thymine dimers and (6-4) photoproducts in DNA by monochromatic ultraviolet light ranging from 150 to 365 nm. *Photochem Photobiol* 1991; 54: 403-10.
6. De Fabo EC, Noonan FP. Mechanism of immunosuppression by ultraviolet irradiation in vivo: evidence for the existence of a unique photoreceptor in the skin and its role in photoimmunology. *J Exp Med* 1983; 157: 84-98.
7. Gibbs NK, Norval M, Traynor NJ, Wolf M, Johnson BE, Crosby J. Action spectra for the trans to cis photoisomerization of urocanic acid in vitro and in mouse skin. *Photochem Photobiol* 1993; 57: 584-90.
8. Kammeyer A, Teunissen MBM, Pavel S, De Rie MA, Bos JD. Photoisomerization spectrum of urocanic acid in human skin and in vitro effects of simulated solar and artificial ultraviolet radiation. *Br J Dermatol* 1995; 132: 884-91.
9. Schauer E, Trautinger F, Köck A, Schwarx A, Bhardwaj R, Simon M, Ansel JC, Schwarz T, Luger TA. Propiomelanocortin-derived peptides are synthesized and released by human keratinocytes. *J Clin Invest* 1994; 83: 2258-62.
10. Wintzen M, Yaar M, Avila EM, Burbach JPH, Gilchrest BA. Propiomelanocortin gene-product regulation in cultured keratinocytes. *J Invest Dermatol* 1996 (in press).
11. Wintzen M, Yaar M, Burbach JPH, Gilchrest BA, Vermeer BJ. Secretion of b endorphin immunoreactivity by cultured human keratinocytes after ultraviolet A radiation. *Abstract J Invest Dermatol* 1996 (in press).
12. De Leeuw SM, Janssen S, Simons JWIM, Lohman PHM, Vermeer BJ, Schothorst AA. The UV action spectra for the clone-forming ability of cultured human melanocytes and keratinocytes. *Photochem Photobiol* 1994; 59: 430-6.

Effects of UVA light on the immune system. A settled issue?

Thomas Schwarz

T. Schwarz: Department of Dermatology, University of Münster, Von Esmarch Strasse 56, D-48149 Münster, Germany.

The adverse effects of UV light on human health include the induction of phototoxicity, premature skin aging, photocarcinogenesis and immunosuppression. While the pathogenic role of UVA in photosensitization and skin aging is well accepted, the contribution of UVA to carcinogenesis and immunosuppression is to date subject of rather controversial discussion. In particular, the effects of UVA light on immune responses have attracted less attention than those mediated by UVB. However, one has to be aware that the vast majority of studies investigating the effects of UV light on immune reactions has been performed using UVB light sources. Probably due to the fact that the initial observations made with UVB were so exciting and important, the focus on UVB continued. Today, it is unanimously accepted that UVB causes immunosuppression and that this effect has important implications for photocarcinogenesis and exacerbation of infectious diseases [1, 2]. In contrast, when asking whether UVA influences the immune system one rather often gets the answer that this is not the case. However, one has to be aware that this answer is based on the fact that just not sufficient data are available. Several studies focusing on the effects of UVB have included UVA experiments just as controls claiming that the same effects could not be achieved with long wave UV [3]. In contrast, those few studies which primarily focused on UVA could show significant effects of long wave UV on the immune system.

While UVA did not suppress contact hypersensitivity, rather high doses suppressed the rejection of highly antigenic tumors transplanted from syngeneic animals, an effect which is similar to that of UVB [4]. Similarly to UVB, UVA significantly reduces the number of Langerhans cells [5]. The depletion of Langerhans cells is regarded to be causally related to the inability to induce contact hypersensitivity by applying haptens on UVB-exposed skin. However, the same dose of UVA which significantly reduced the number of Langerhans cells did not impair the induction of contact hypersensitivity indicating that a further mechanism besides Langerhans cell depletion might be important for the suppression of the induction of CHS. Accordingly, Baadsgaard *et al.* [5] observed that as a consequence of UVB exposure DR^+CD1^- cells migrate into the epidermis. Subsequent studies showed that these immigrating macrophage like cells are responsible for the induction of hapten-specific suppressor cells which ultimately inhibit sensitization. These DR^+CD1^- epidermal cells are absent in control skin, but are found induced both by UVB and UVC. In contrast, UVA, despite the usage of more than 1,200 times greater doses than for UVB and UVC, UVA was a poor inducer of these cells. Thus, the UV wavelengths for inducing DR^+CD1^- cells lie predominantly within the UVB, and not in the UVA range explaining why UVA does not inhibit the induction of contact hypersensitivity. The wavelenghts appear to be analogous to both the wavelengths for generation of increased host susceptibility to UV-induced murine tumors and to the wavelengths for UV-induced systemic suppression of CHS. Because of the observation that the UV wavelengths which decrease the number of Langerhans cells differ from the wavelengths which suppress of contact hypersensitivity, the appearance of DR^+CD1^- epidermal cells, but not the disappearance of DR^+CD1^+ Langerhans cells, appears to be related to the induction of antigen-specific suppressor cells.

Sjöval and Christensen [6] showed that UVB suppressed both locally and systemically, human allergic contact dermatitis, while UVA had no such effect. However, in this study the UVA dose applied was below 20 J/cm^2. In terms of UVA effectiveness, this is not a high dose and thus the only permissible conclusion is that UVA at such low doses has no effect. Repetition of these studies with higher doses up to 100 J/cm^2 are eagerly awaited. This request is also based on *in vitro* studies. Pretell *et al.* [7] observed that UV radiation of hapten-conjugated stimulator cells inhibits the proliferative T cell response. Surprisingly, not only UVB but also UVA irradiation turned out to be suppressive. Fifty percent inhibition was already observed after application of 10 J/cm^2. The inhibition was significantly greater if UV radiation followed haptenation rather than preceeding it. There is also *in vivo* evidence that UVA can affect the immune system. The famous study by Hersey *et al.* [8] addressing immunological changes induced by solarium exposure is mostly quoted when referring to the immunosuppressive effects of UVB. However, one has to be aware that the UV device used emitted mostly UVA and only minimal UVB. A follow-up study could clearly show that the inhibitory effect on natural killer cells was mainly due to the UVA range [9]. Groups of volunteers were exposed to solarium radiation that was filtered through a Mylar sheeting which absorbs UVB. Natural killer cell activity was depressed in the group exposed to radiation and this was not prevented by filtration through the Mylar filter. UVB filtering, however, appeared to prevent changes in blood lymphocyte subsets that are induced by solarium radiation as well as the reduction in Langerhans cell numbers in skin biopsies taken after exposure to solarium radiation.

Recently, the UVA spectrum has been separated arbitrarily into a short wave range (320-340 nm), called UVA2, and a long wave range (340-400 nm), called UVA1. Being aware of the well known immunosuppressive properties of UVB light, it was anticipated that immunosuppressive effects of UVA may be more pronounced in the UVA2 than in the UVA1 range. This may be true, but it has however, led to the unjustified conclusion that UVA1 does not affect the immune system at all and thus can be regarded as harmless and thus safe. Of course, one has to admit that insufficient studies addressing the immunomodulatory effects of UVA1 are available to date. However, there is accumulating evidence that UVA1 does have an effect on the immune system, *e.g.*, exposure of long-term cultured human keratinocytes to UVB or to UVA1 radiation caused a time and dose dependent induction of IL-10 mRNA expression and IL-10 protein secretion [10]. Interestingly, the UVA1 range turned out to be a significantly stronger stimulus than UVB. Since IL-10 inhibits the cytokine secretion by T helper 1 cells and interferes with antigen presentation IL-10 has been recognized as a cytokine with immunosuppressive properties. UVA1 therapy was recently found to be superior to UVB radiation in the treatment of atopic dermatitis, and the clinical improvement induced by UVA1 appeared to be due to reduction of lesional IFN γ expression in atopic eczema [11]. It is therefore tempting to speculate that UVA1-induced expression of IL-10 by keratinocytes accounts, at least in part, for downregulation of T helper 1 cell derived cytokines in inflammatory skin diseases. Moreover, it was recently observed that exposure of human keratinocytes to UVA1 light induces the expression of the adhesion molecule ICAM-1 as was observed with UVB. Analysis of the underlying mechanism, however, indicates that UVA1 and UVB induce ICAM-1 *via* different pathways.

UVA light also plays an important role in photoageing *via* the release of cytokines. Accordingly, it has been shown that UVA reaches the reticular dermis making fibroblasts an accessible target, inducing the release of collagenase by fibroblasts. Since IL-6 stimulates collagenase production by fibroblasts, the relation between the UV-induced collagenase increase and IL-6 was studied [12]. Confluent fibroblast layers exposed to UVA1-light released significantly enhanced levels of IL-6 which was also confirmed by Northern blot analysis. Incubation of irradiated cells with IL-6 antisense oligonucleotides resulted in a significant, but not complete downregulation of collagenase. The failure of complete blocking may be due to the fact that UVA-induced release of other mediators such as IL-1 by fibroblasts is involved in the induction of collagenase as well [12].

Taken together, the effects of UVA light on the immune system are far from being completely understood. To evaluate the health risk of UVA light, additional studies addressing these issues are urgently needed. Without these studies, it is premature to claim that UVA light does not affect the immune system.

References

1. Kripke ML. Immunology and photocarcinogenesis. New light on an old problem. *J Am Acad Dermatol* 1986; 14: 149-55.
2. Chapman RS, Cooper KD, DeFabo EC, Frederick JE, Gelatt KN, Hammond SP, Hersey P, Koren HS, Ley RD, Noonan F, Rusch GM, Sarasin A, Selgrade MJ, Sobolev I, Ward BK, Werkema TE. Solar ultraviolet radiation and the risk of infectious disease. *Photochem Photobiol* 1994; 61: 223-47.
3. Kirnbauer R, Köck A, Neuner P, Förster E, Krutmann J, Urbanski A, Schauer E, Ansel JC, Schwarz T, Luger TA. Regulation of epidermal cell interleukin 6 production by UV light and corticosteroids. *J Invest Dermatol* 1991; 96: 484-9.
4. Gange RW, Rosen CF. UVA effects on mammalian skin and cells. *Photochem Photobiol* 1986; 43: 701-5.
5. Baadsgaard O, Wulf HC, Lange Wantzin G, Cooper KD. UVB and UVC, but not UVA, potently induce the appearance of T6–DR+ antigen-presenting cells in human epidermis. *J Invest Dermatol* 1987; 89: 113-8.
6. Sjöval P, Christensen OB. Local and systemic effect of ultraviolet irradiation (UVB and UVA) on human allergic contact dermatitis. *Acta Derm Venereol* 1986; 66: 290-4.
7. Pretell JO, McAuliffe DJ, Parrish JA. Ultraviolet radiation inhibits both accessory cell and responder T cell function in the proliferative response to haptenated-self. *Photochem Photobiol* 1984; 40: 337-42.
8. Hersey P, Bradley M, Hasic E, Haran G, Edwards A, McCarthy WH. Immunological effects of solarium exposure. *Lancet* 1983; i: 545-8.
9. Hersey P, Mac Donald M, Henderson C, Schibeci S, D'Alessandro G, Pryor M, Wilkinson FJ. Suppression of natural killer cell activity in humans by radiation from solarium lamps depleted of UVB. *J Invest Dermatol* 1988; 90: 305-10.
10. Grewe M, Gyufko K, Krutmann J. Interleukin 10: production by cultured human keratinocytes: regulation by ultraviolet B and ultraviolet A1 radiation. *J Invest Dermatol* 1995; 104: 3-6.
11. Krutmann J, Czech W, Diepgen T, Niedner R, Kapp A, Schöpf E. High-dose UVA1 therapy in the treatment of patients with atopic dermatitis. *J Am Acad Dermatol* 1992; 26: 225-30.
12. Wlaschek M, Bolsen K, Herrmann G, Schwarz A, Wilmroth F, Heinrich PC, Goerz G, Scharffetter-Kochanek K. UVA-induced autocrine stimulation of fibroblast-derived collagenase by IL-6: a possible mechanism in dermal photodamage? *J Invest Dermatol* 1993; 101: 164-8.

Ultraviolet A radiation-induced immunomodulation: molecular and photobiological mechanisms

Jean Krutmann

J. Krutmann: Department of Dermatology, Heinrich-Heine-University, Moorenstr. 5, D-40225 Düsseldorf, Germany.

Solar UVA radiation contributes to photoageing and photocarcinogenesis of human skin and is responsible for triggering the most frequent photodermatoses, *i.e.* polymorphous light eruption [1]. Human skin is additionally exposed to UVA radiation from artificial sources including high-intensity UVA irradiation devices, which in former years have mainly been used for cosmetical purposes, but are currently employed at an increasing rate for the treatment of inflammatory skin diseases such as atopic dermatitis, urticaria pigmentosa and connective tissue diseases [2-5]. The detrimental and beneficial effects of UVA radiation are at least partially due to its capacity to modulate the expression of immunologically relevant genes in, and thereby the immune function of, human skin cells. For example, UVA radiation is a potent inducer of the immunosuppressive cytokine, interleukin (IL)-10 in human keratinocytes and upregulates FAS-ligand gene expression in skin-infiltrating T-cells, thereby leading to T-cell apoptosis. From a phototherapeutical point of view, these two effects are antiinflammatory and responsible for the therapeutic effectiveness of UVA radiation phototherapy in the treatment of patients with T cell-mediated, inflammatory skin diseases [5, 6]. Induction of proinflammatory gene expression in keratinocytes of patients with polymorphous light eruption, on the other hand, constitutes a detrimental effect that contributes to the development of skin lesions in UVA-exposed skin areas of these patients. In order to better understand UVA radiation-induced immunomodulatory effects it is necessary to analyse the photobiological and molecular mechanisms responsible for UVA radiation-induced gene regulation.

These studies are of particular interest, because biological effects induced by short wavelength and long wavelength UV radiation involve different chromophores leading to different photobiological effects [7]. It is therefore likely that the mechanisms by which UVA radiation induces transcriptional activation of human genes differ from those induced by UVC or UVB radiation. Recent studies from our group support this concept and indicate the existence of a unique and previously unrecognized signal transduction pathway, by which UVA radiation induces gene expression in human keratinocytes. This pathway appears to be mediated through the generation of singlet oxygen and to involve activator protein-2 (AP-2) [8].

Photobiological aspects of UVA radiation-induced gene expression

The growing list of UVA radiation-inducible genes includes the heme-oxygenase-1 gene (HO-1), various cytokines, the adhesion molecule intercellular adhesion molecule-1 (ICAM-1), matrix meltalloproteinases, the FAS-ligand molecule (CD95-L), and CL100, a non-receptor-type protein-tyrosine phosphatase. Ultraviolet A radiation-induced expression of the HO-1, MMP-1, ICAM-1, FAS-L, and possibly also selected cytokine genes involve the generation of reactive oxygen species [9, 10]. In transformed human keratinocytes, UVA radiation-induced ICAM-1 expression was only observed in cells that had been pretreated with an inhibitor of *de novo* glutathione synthesis, indicating that UVA radiation-induced ICAM-1 expression occurred through a mechanism which depended on the thiol-status of the irradiated cells [10, 11]. This effect was specific for UVA radiation-induced ICAM-1 expression, because UVB radiation increased ICAM-1 gene expression regardless of whether these cells had been depleted of endogenous glutathione or not. A similar induction pattern was also observed for selected cytokine genes including interleukin (IL)-1α and IL-6 [11].

The observation that UVA radiation-induced ICAM-1 expression in human keratinocytes is modulated through cellular glutathione levels points to a prominent role of reactive oxygen species (ROIs) in this system. Induction of the HO-1 gene in UVA-irradiated human dermal fibroblasts was efficiently blocked by singlet oxygen quenchers such as sodium azide and L-histidine, it was enhanced if the cells were irradiated in the presence of deuterium oxide in which singlet oxygen has a longer half-life, and it was mimicked upon stimulation with Rose Bengal plus light, a known singlet oxygen generating system [12]. These data indicated that singlet oxygen generation is important for UVA radiation-induced gene expression. This conclusion was corroborated and extended in subsequent studies in which singlet oxygen was found to mediate UVA radiation-induced MMP-1 expression in human dermal fibroblasts [13], UVA radiation-induced ICAM-1 expression in human epidermal keratinocytes [14], and UVA radiation-induced FAS-L upregulation in skin-infiltrating human T-helper cells [6]. Singlet oxygen thus seems to be the primary effector in UVA radiation-induced gene expression. Analysis of the molecular mechanisms involved in UVA-induced gene expression have therefore also provided insight into the mechanisms by which singlet oxygen activates transcription factors and induces promotor activation.

Molecular aspects of UVA radiation-induced gene expression

Ultraviolet A radiation and singlet oxygen-induced promoter activation have recently been studied by using promoter constructs based on the human ICAM-1 promoter [14]. Both stimuli were found to activate transcription factor AP-2, and deletion of the putative AP-2 binding site abrogated ICAM-1 promoter activation in UVA-irradiated or singlet oxygen-stimulated human keratinocytes. It has therefore been concluded that the AP-2 site served as both the UVA-responsive and the singlet-responsive element of the human ICAM-1 gene. Deletion of the AP-2 site did not abrogate UVB radiation-induced ICAM-1 promoter activation, indicating that UVB radiation- and UVA radiation-induced gene expression do not only differ with regard to the photobiological mechanisms involved, but also depend on different molecular mechanisms [8, 14]. The critical role of AP-2 in UVA radiation-induced gene expression is further emphasized by very recent studies, in which the functional role of AP-2 and its alternative splice product AP-2B was studied for UVA radiation-induced gene expression. AP-2B results from alternative usage of exon 5 and differs from AP-2 in the C-terminus [15]. It lacks the dimerization domain required for DNA binding, but contains the transactivation domain and part of the DNA-binding domain [16]. Studies addressing the functional relevance of AP-2B have revealed that it serves as a dominant negative regulator of AP-2 transactivation [16, 17]. This concept is in line with the recent observation that in UVA-irradiated human epidermal keratinocytes, increased ICAM-1 expression was always observed at time points when the ratio of AP-2/AP-2B was shifted towards AP-2 [18]. Similarly, cells that had been stably transfected to overexpress AP-2 [16] showed a 1,000-fold increase ICAM-1 expression, as compared to the parental clone, whereas AP-2B overexpression was associated with a failure of cells to upregulate ICAM-1 expression above baseline levels following UVA irradiation [18]. Preliminary data imply that this pattern of UVA radiation-induced gene expression in AP-2 *versus* AP-2B overexpressing cells is not specific for ICAM-1, but may be observed for other UVA radiation- and possibly also singlet oxygen-inducible genes as well. The promoter regions of almost all of these genes contain one or several putative AP-2 binding sites, which in case of the HO-1 gene share a strong homology to the AP-2 site present in the human ICAM-1 promoter [8]. Based on this information it is tempting to speculate that activation of transcription factor AP-2 may constitute a general mechanism by which UVA radiation and/or singlet oxygen induce gene expression in human keratinocytes.

Ceramide signaling and ultraviolet A radiation (UVAR)-induced gene expression

Recent studies indicate that ceramides are part of the signal transduction pathway operative in UVA radiation-induced, AP-2 mediated gene expression [19]. By employing gel electrophoretic-mobility shift assays we have observed that treatment of KC with ceramides increased DNA-binding activity of transcription factor AP-2. In order to assess the functional relevance of ceramide-induced AP-2 activation, KC were transiently transfected with a series of ICAM-1 based luciferase reporter gene constructs. Constructs with ICAM-1 fragments up to 6,000/+ 1 displayed significant responsiveness to stimulation with UVA radiation or ceramide. For both stimuli, responsiveness was completely abolished, if a construct lacking the AP-2 site was used, indicating a cause-effect relationship. Accordingly, exposure to UVA radiation significantly (3-fold) increased the formation of ceramides in human keratinocytes. Moreover, UVAR-induced ICAM-1 mRNA expression in KC could be completely prevented by treatment of cells with cycloserine or fumonisin B, which both inhibit ceramide synthesis, but at different levels. These effects were specific, because addition of ceramides to inhibitor-treated KC post-irradiation restored ICAM-1 expression, and because these inhibitors did not prevent cytokine (TNFα, IFN-γ)-induced KC ICAM-1 expression. Ceramides thus play a previously unrecognized role in AP-2 activation and UVA radiation-induced gene expression.

Concluding remarks

If our interpretation of the data is correct, the results would imply that AP-2 activation is of general importance for UVA radiation-induced gene expression. We therefore propose that AP-2 activation represents a defined biological endpoint to measure UVA radiation-induced effects as they relate to photodermatoses, photoageing and photocarcinogenesis.

References

1. Urbach F, ed. *Biological responses to ultraviolet A radiation*. Valdenmar, Overland Park, Kansas, 1992.
2. Krutmann J. High-dose UVA1 therapy for inflammatory skin disease. *Dermatol Ther* 1997; 4: 123-8.
3. Stege H, Humke S, Berneburg M, Dierks K, Goerz G, Ruzicka T, Krutmann J. High-dose UVA1 therapy in the treatment of patients with localized scleroderma. *J Am Acad Dermatol* 1997; 36: 938-44.
4. Stege H, Schöpf E, Ruzicka T, Krutmann J. High-dose UVA1 for urticaria pigmentosa. *Lancet* 1996; 347: 64.
5. Krutmann J. Therapeutic photomedicine : phototherapy. In: *Fitzpatrick's Dermatology in General Medicine*. 5th edition. Freedberg IM, Eisen AB, Wolff K, Austen KF, Goldsmith LA, Katz SI, Fitzpatrick TB, eds. McGraw-Hill, New York, 1998.
6. Morita A, Werfel T, Stege H, Ahrens C, Grewe M, Grether-Beck S, Ruzicka T, Kapp A, Klotz LO, Sies H, Krutmann J. Evidence that singlet oxygen-induced human T-helper cell apoptosis is the basic mechanism of ultraviolet-A radiation phototherapy. *J Exp Med* 1997; 186: 1763-8.
7. Kochevar IE. Primary processes in photobiology and photosensitation. In: *Photoimmunology*. Krutmann J, Elmets CA, eds. Blackwell Science Ltd, 1995: 19-33.
8. Grether-Beck S, Buettner R, Krutmann J. Ultraviolet A radiation-induced expression of human genes: molecular and photobiological mechanisms. *Biol Chem* 1997; 378: 1231-6.
9. Tyrrell RM. Activation of mammalian gene expression by the UV component of sunlight – from models to reality. *Bioassays* 1996; 18: 139-48.
10. Krutmann J, Grewe M. Involvement of cytokines, DNA damage, and reactive oxygen intermediates in ultraviolet radiation-induced modulation of intercellular adhesion molecule-1 (ICAM-1) expression. *J Invest Dermatol* 1995; 105: 67S-70S.
11. Morita A, Grewe M, Grether-Beck S, Olaizola-Horn S, Krutmann J. Induction of proinflammatory cytokines in human epidermoid carcinoma cells by in vitro ultraviolet A1 irradiation. *Photochem Photobiol* 1997; 65: 630-5.
12. Basu-Modak S, Tyrrell RM. Singlet oxygen: a primary effector in the ultraviolet A/near-visible light induction of the human heme oxygenase gene. *Cancer Res* 1993; 53: 4505-19.
13. Wlaschek M, Brivida K, Stricklin GP, Sies H, Scharfetter-Kochanek K. Singlet oxygen may mediate the ultraviolet A-induced synthesis of interstitial collagenase. *J Invest Dermatol* 1995; 104: 194-8.
14. Grether-Beck S, Olaizola-Horn S, Schmitt H, Grewe M, Jahnke A, Johnson JP, Brivida K, Sies H, Krutmann J. Activation of transcription factor AP-2 mediates UVA radiation- and singlet oxygen-induced expression of the human intercellular adhesion molecule 1 gene. *Proc Natl Acad Sci USA* 1996; 93: 14586-91.
15. Bauer R, Imhof A, Pscherer A, Kopp H, Moser M, Seegers S, Kerscher M, Tainky MA, Hofstaedter F, Buettner R. The genomic structure of the human AP-2 transcription factor. *Nucl Acids Res* 1994; 22: 1413-20.
16. Buettner R, Kannan P, Imhof A, Bauer R, Yim SO, Glockshuber R, van Dyke MW, Tainsky MA. An alternatively spliced mRNA from the AP-2 gene encodes a negative regulator of transcriptional activation by AP-2. *Mol Cell Biol* 1993; 13: 4174-85.

17. Duan C, Clemmons DR. Transcription factor AP-2 regulates human insulin-like growth factor binding protein-5 gene expression. *J Biol Chem* 1995; 270: 24844-51.
18. Grether-Beck S, Schmitt H, Grewe M, Buettner R, Krutmann J. The balance between expression of transcription factor AP2 and its alternative splice product AP2B controls ultraviolet A radiation (UVAR)-induced gene expression in human cells. Abstract. *J Invest Dermatol* 1997; 108: 594.
19. Grether-Beck S, Schmitt H, Felsner I, Bonizzi G, Piette J, Johnson JP, Klotz LO, Krutmann J. Ceramide signaling is a key component of ultraviolet A radiation-induced gene expression in human keratinocytes. Abstract. *J Invest Dermatol* 1998; in press.

UVA1 radiation-induced immunomodulatory and gene regulatory effects in human keratinocytes

Jean Krutmann

J. Krutmann: Department of Dermatology, Heinrich-Heine-University, Moorenstrasse 5, D-40225, Düsseldorf, Germany.

Ultraviolet radiation (UVR)-induced modulation of the immune function of epidermal keratinocytes is thought to be important for the pathogenesis of photosensitive skin diseases such as polymorphous light eruption [1]. This is consistent with recent observations of an increased expression of keratinocyte-derived proinflammatory cytokines (IL-1, IL-8) and adhesion molecules (ICAM-1) in lesional skin of patients with polymorphous light eruption [2, 3]. In previous years, extensive research has focused on studying the effects of ultraviolet B radiation (UVBR; 280-315 nm) on keratinocyte expression of immunomodulatory cytokines and adhesion molecules [4], although ultraviolet A1 radiation (UVA1R; 340-400 nm) rather than UVBR is a more frequent trigger of polymorphous light eruption [1]. There is also increasing evidence that UVA1R may be effectively used in the phototherapy of inflammatory/immunologically-based skin diseases [5]. Exposure of human skin to high-doses of UVA1R (high-dose UVA1 therapy) has been found to be highly effective in the management of patients with severe atopic dermatitis [6, 7], and preliminary studies indicate that this modality may also be of benefit for patients with urticaria pigmentosa [8] and localized scleroderma [9]. In aggregate these studies imply that UVA1R, similarily to UVBR, has the capacity to exert immunomodulatory effects on the skin immune system. It was therefore not surprising to learn that UVA1R is able to induce synthesis and release of anti- as well as proinflammatory cytokines from human epidermal keratinocytes and to affect adhesion molecule expression in these cells. Recent studies have also advanced our knowledge about the photobiological and molecular mechanisms which are responsible for UVA1R-induced immunomodulatory effects, which were found to differ from those identified for UVBR-induced immunomodulation. This review will provide a brief summary of our studies on UVA1R-induced modulation of keratinocyte cytokine and adhesion molecule expression with particular emphasis on the underlying gene regulatory mechanisms.

Ultraviolet A1 radiation effects on keratinocyte immune function

The first cytokine that has been reported to be markedly induced upon exposure of normal human keratinocytes to UVA1R is the anti-inflammatory cytokine interleukin IL-10 [10].

UVA1R did not only increase the release of IL-10 protein into supernatants of irradiated keratinocytes, but also markedly enhanced steady state levels of IL-10 specific mRNA within these cells, indicating that UVA1R-induced keratinocyte IL-10 production was caused by UVA1R-induced synthesis of this immunomodulatory molecule. The capacity of UVA1R to affect keratinocyte cytokine expression is not restricted to IL-10. Recent studies at our laboratory have demonstrated that in addition to IL-10, increased mRNA and protein expression of TNFα, IL-1α, IL-6 and IL-8 may be observed in UVA1-irradiated keratinocytes [11]. In these experiments, cells from the human epidermoid carcinoma cell line KB rather than normal human keratinocytes were employed, which differ from normal keratinocytes by exhibiting significantly higher (app. 4-fold) levels of endogenous glutathione. It is important to note that increased expression of IL-1α and IL-6 could only be observed in UVA1-irradiated KB cells, if their endogenous glutathione content was decreased prior to UVA1R exposure. In contrast, expression and release of TNFα and IL-8 was induced in UVA1-irradiated KB cells regardless of their endogenous glutathione levels. These experiments indicate that thiol status-dependent (IL-1α, IL-6) and independent (IL-8, TNFα) mechanisms are involved in UVA1R-induced modulation of human keratinocyte cytokine expression.

This assumption was further supported by studies in which expression of the adhesion molecule ICAM-1 was analyzed in UVA1-irradiated normal human keratinocytes as well as KB cells [12, 13]. We observed that UVA1R was very well capable of inducing ICAM-1 mRNA and surface expression in normal keratinocytes, but only weak or no upregulation could be observed in KB cells. If, however, KB cells were glutathione depleted prior to UVA1 irradiation, upregulation of ICAM-1 expression was seen to an extent identical to that observed for normal keratinocytes. Further analysis of the underlying photobiological mechanism revealed that the generation of reactive oxygen species (ROS) was important for UVA1R-induced keratinocytes ICAM-1 expression. Pretreatment of cells with the antioxidant vitamin E or irradiation of cells in the presence of the singlet oxygen quencher sodium acide completely inhibited UVA1R-induced ICAM-1 expression, and UVA1R exposure of cells in the presence of deuterium oxide, which increases the half-life of singlet oxygen, was found to significantly enhance UVA1R-induced ICAM-1 expression. The effects of vitamin E, sodium acide and deuterium oxide were specific for UVA1-induced ICAM-1 expression, since they could not be observed for UVBR-induced ICAM-1 expression. These studies suggest that UVA1R-induced upregulation of keratinocyte ICAM-1 expression is mediated by an oxidative mechanism which appears to involve the generation of singlet oxygen [13, 14].

Ultraviolet A1 radiation-induced gene regulatory effects

We have recently asked whether different gene regulatory mechanisms may be involved in UVA1R- *versus* UVBR-induced immunomodulation of human keratinocytes. In these studies, human keratinocytes were transiently transfected with a series of ICAM-1 based luciferase reporter gene constructs [15]. We have found that constructs with the ICAM-1 fragments up to 6,000/+1 displayed significant responsiveness to UVA1R, which was not inhibited by deletion of binding sites for NFkB or AP-1, but was completely abolished, if a construct lacking the AP-2 binding site was used. Deletion of the AP-2 binding site specifically inhibited UVA1R-induced ICAM-1 promotor activation, since it did not inhibit UVBR or IL-1α-induced-ICAM-1 based reporter gene activity. The role of AP-2 in UVA1R-induced keratinocyte gene activation was further supported by gel retardation mobility shift assays demonstrating increased activation of AP-2 in nuclear extracts isolated from UVA1-irradiated cells. Most interestingly, stimulation of non-irradiated keratinocytes with the singlet oxygen generating system $NDPO_2$ induced ICAM-1 promotor activation comparable to that achieved by UVA1R, and $NDPO_2$-induced ICAM-1 promotor activation was abolished upon deletion of the AP-2 binding site. These studies demonstrate that the AP-2 binding site of the ICAM-1 gene serves as both the UVA1R- and singlet oxygen responsive element, indicating a cause/effect relationship.

Conclusion

Our studies clearly indicate that similar to UVBR, UVA1R has the capacity to affect the immune function of epidermal keratinocytes by modulating cytokine and adhesion molecule expression. The photobiological and gene regulatory mechanisms underlying UVA1R-induced immunomodulation, however, differ from those involved in UVBR-induced immunomodulation. In addition, there is a growing body of evidence that UVA1R-induced immunomodulation is not restricted to epidermal keratinocytes, but clearly extends to epidermal as well as dermal dendritic cells, dermal mast cells [16], and skin-infiltrating T cells [17, 18]. Future research on the immunomodulatory capacities of UVA1R will not only provide important insight into the pathogenesis of UVA-sensitive photodermatoses such as polymorphous light eruption and the relevance of UVA radiation to photocarcinogenesis, it may also help to develop efficient strategies for the protection of human skin against harmful effects associated with UVA radiation. In addition, these studies may stimulate improvement and further development of UVA radiation therapy and, in particular, UVA1R phototherapy of skin diseases.

References

1. Norris PG. Advances in understanding the pathogenesis of photodermatosis. *Curr Op Dermatol* 1993; 1: 185-90.
2. Norris P, Morris J, McGibbon DH, Chu AC, Hawk JLM. Polymorphous light eruption: an immunopathological study of evolving lesions. *Br J Dermatol* 1989; 120: 173-83.
3. Norris P, Bacon K, Bird C, Hawk J, Camp RL. Lymphocyte attractant activity in suction blister samples from polymorphous light eruption and chronic actinic dermatitis. *Br J Dermatol* 1991; 125: 484.
4. Krutmann J, Elmets CA. *Photoimmunology*. Oxford: Blackwell Science Ltd, 1995.
5. Krutmann J. Ultraviolet A1 radiation-induced immunomodulation: high-dose UVA1 therapy of atopic dermatitis. In: *Photoimmunology*. Krutman J, Elmets CA, eds. Oxford: Blackwell Science Ltd, 1995; 246-56.
6. Krutmann J, Czech W, Diepgen T, Niedner T, Kapp A, Schöpf E. High-dose UVA1 therapy in the treatment of patients with atopic dermatitis. *J Am Acad Dermatol* 1992; 26: 225-30.
7. Krutmann J, Diepgen T, Luger TA, Grabbe S, Meffert H, Sönnichsen N, Czech W, Kapp A, Stege H, Grewe M, Schöpf E. High-dose UVA1 therapy for atopic dermatitis: a multicenter trial. *J Invest Dermatol* 1995; 105: 45A.
8. Stege H, Schöpf E, Ruzicka T, Krutmann J. High-dose UVA1 for urticaria pigmentosa. *Lancet* 1996; 347: 64.

9. Stege H, Humke S, Berneburg M, Dierks K, Müller-Forte S, Goerz G, Ruzicka T, Krutmann J. High-dose UVA1 therapy in the treatment of patients with localized scleroderma. Abstract *J Invest Dermatol* 1996 (in press).
10. Grewe M, Gyufko K, Krutmann J. Interleukin-10 production by cultured human keratinocytes: regulation by ultraviolet B and A1 radiation. *J Invest Dermatol* 1995; 104: 3-6.
11. Morita A, Grewe M, Ahrens C, Grether-Beck S, Ruzicka T, Krutmann J. Ultraviolet A1 radiation effects on cytokine expression in human epidermoid carcinoma cells. *Photochem Photobiol* 1996 (in press).
12. Christoph H, Parlow F, Budnik A, Block R, Schöpf E, Krutmann J. Ultraviolet A1 radiation-induced immunomodulation: UVA1- and UVB-radiation both affect human keratinocyte expression of intercellular adhesion molecule-1 (ICAM-1), although by different mechanisms. Abstract *Arch Dermatol Res* 1993; 285: 56.
13. Olaizola-Horn S, Christoph H, Budnik A, Grewe M, Grether-Beck S, Gyufko K, Luscher P, Tyrrell RM, Krutmann J. Ultraviolet A1 radiation-induced upregulation of keratinocyte expression of intercellular adhesion molecule-1 (ICAM-1) is mediated via the generation of free radicals. Abstract *Arch Dermatol Res* 1993; 286: 38.
14. Krutmann J, Grewe M. Involvement of cytokines, DNA damage, and reactive oxygen intermediates in ultraviolet radiation-induced modulation of intercellular adhesion molecule-1 expression. *J Invest Dermatol* 1995; 105: 67S-70S.
15. Grether-Beck S, Schmitt H, Grewe M, Jahnke A, Johnson JP, Briviba K, Sies H, Krutmann J. The ultraviolet A1 radiation-responsive and the singlet oxygen responsive element of the human ICAM-1 gene may be identical. Abstract *Arch Dermatol Res* 1996 (in press).
16. Grabbe J, Welker P, Humke S, Grewe M, Schöpf E, Henz BM, Krutmann J. Differential effects of high-dose UVA1 therapy versus UVA/UVB therapy on IgE binding cells in lesional skin of patients with atopic eczema. *J Invest Dermatol* 1996 (in press).
17. Grewe M, Gyufko K, Schöpf E, Krutmann J. Lesional expression of interferon-g in atopic eczema. *Lancet* 1994; 343: 23-5.
18. Morita A, Grewe M, Werfel T, Kapp A, Krutmann J. Ultraviolet A1 radiation differentially affects cytokine production by atopen-specific human T-helper cells. Abstract *J Invest Dermatol* 1996 (in press).

Immunomodulation by UV light: role of neuropeptides

Thomas A. Luger

T.A. Luger: Ludwig Boltzmann Institute for Cell Biology and Immunobiology of the Skin, Department of Dermatology, University of Münster, Münster, Germany.

Exposure of the skin to ultraviolet (UV) radiation is well known to result in profound alterations of the local as well as the systemic immune response and to cause skin cancer. Although, UV directly affects the function of epidermal cell including melanocytes, keratinocytes and Langerhans cells, many of its effects are mediated *via* the induction of soluble mediators [1]. In addition to cytokines, neuropeptides were recently found to be produced by many different cells including epithelial and inflammatory cells and to be part of the network of mediators regulating immune and inflammatory reactions [2].

Among several neuropeptides such as substance P, vasointestinal peptide, calcitonin gene-related peptide a.o. keratinocytes recently have been shown to produce proopiomelanocortin (POMC), which is the precursor for adrenocorticotrophin (ACTH), β-endorphin (β-E), β-lipotrophic hormone (β-LPH) and the melanocyte-stimulating hormones (α, β, and γ MSH). The POMC precursor undergoes cleavage *via* the proteolytic activities of a family of prohormone-converting enzymes (PC) which were also found to be expressed in keratinocytes [3]. POMC-peptides exert their multiple activities *via* a group of 5 G-protein-coupled receptors, which have been designated as melanocortin receptor (MC) 1R-5R. MC1-R is specific for αMSH and ACTH, it shows the widest distribution and was recently found to be expressed on keratinocytes as well as immunocompetent cells [3, 4].

Effect of UV-light on melanocortins in the skin

POMC-peptides have been detected in many cells of the skin including melanocytes, keratinocytes, Langerhans cells, endothelial cells, and fibroblasts [3, 5]. Moreover, epidermal as well as dermal cells are not only a source but also a target for POMC-peptides [3, 4]. Keratinocytes are known to produce a wide variety of mediators such as cytokines, chemokines, growth factors, eicosanoides, lipoproteins and parahormone-like proteins [6]. In addition, normal as well as malignant keratinocytes express POMC mRNA and release αMSH, ACTH and β-endorphin. Without stimulation, only low amounts of POMC-peptides are detectable in normal human skin, but upon treatment with tumor promoters (PMA) or IL-1, a significant upregulation of POMC mRNA expression and POMC-peptides release has been observed [3]. In addition, irradiation of keratinocytes with UVB (25 mJ/cm^2) or UVA1 (10 J/m^2) significantly enhanced the expression of POMC-specific mRNA as well as the release of αMSH [7]. To control the production of these peptides, tissue-specific prohormone convertases are required, which recently have been detected in keratinocytes. Accordingly, keratinocytes *in vitro* express PC-1 mRNA which was upregulated upon UVB (25 mJ/cm^2) irradiation. Thus, UV exposure seems to modulate POMC-peptide production both at the transcriptional as well as the posttranslational level [8].

Among the various melanocortin receptors only MC-1h has been detected in normal as well as transformed human keratinocytes [9]. Treatment of keratinocytes with UVB (25 mJ/cm^2) was able to upregulate MC-1R mRNA expression as well as the binding of labeled αMSH, suggesting that UV irradiation stimulates the expression of a functional αMSH receptor on keratinocytes [8]. Accordingly, αMSH is capable of enhancing keratinocyte proliferation, downregulates the expression of heat shock proteins (HSP70) in keratinocytes and renders them more sensitive to oxidative stress [10].

Immunomodulating effects of POMC-peptides

POMC-peptides such as αMSH affect immune and inflammatory reactions in several ways. The function and production of proinflammatory and immunomodulating cytokines such as IL-α, IL-β, IL-6, TNFα, IL-2 and IFNγ are antagonized by αMSH, and it also inhibits fever, leukocytosis, release of acute phase proteins, IL-2 receptor expression as well as neutrophil chemotaxis [3, 11]. The immunosuppressing function of αMSH was supported by a recent study showing that αMSH upregulates IL-10 expression in human peripheral blood monocytes [12]. Since IL-10 is a potent inhibitor immunomodulating cytokine synthesis and *in vivo* downregulates contact hypersensitivity (CHS) as well as delayed type hypersensitivity (DTH) responses, the immunosuppressive effects of αMSH appear to occur at least in part *via* IL-10 induction [13]. This is further supported by the finding that in the murine system, administration of αMSH blocks the induction as well as elicitation of CHS and causes hapten- specific tolerance [14]. Since UV-light has been shown to upregulate IL-10 and αMSH production *in vivo* as well as *in vitro*, these mediators, *via* the downregulation of costimulatory signals such as IL-1, IL-12, CD40 and CD86, may function as crucial mediators of UV-induced immunosuppression and tolerance induction [3].

There is evidence that among immunocompetent cells the major target for αMSH are monocytes. Thus, monocytes, macrophages and monocytic cell lines have been shown to express receptors specific for POMC-peptides [15, 16]. The expression of MC1-R by monocytes is enhanced upon treatment with mitogens or lectins and was also found to be upregulated during the activation and maturation of monocytes [15]. In addition to immunocompetent cells, human dermal microvascular endothelial cells which play a crucial role in early steps of any immune and inflammatory response were found to express MC1-R [17]. Upon treatment of endothelial cells with αMSH, the LPS-induced expression of adhesion molecules such as VCAM and E-selectin was downregulated in a dose-dependent manner. Moreover, the LPS-mediated activation of transcription factors such as NFκB and cyclic AMP responsive binding protein (CRAP) was inhibited by αMSH [18]. Since several adhesion molecules including VCAM and E-selectin contain regulatory NFκB sites in their promoter regions and PC1 expression is under the control of CRAP, many of the immunomodulating effects of αMSH seem to be due to its effect on the activation of transcription factor.

These findings indicate that POMC-peptides such as αMSH are produced in the skin upon UV-irradiation and by modulating the function of antigen-presenting cells and dermal microvascular endothelial cells appear to play a crucial role in UV-mediated immunosuppression. Further studies will determine whether application of αMSH or one of its peptides may be useful for the treatment of inflammatory, allergic or autoimmune diseases.

Acknowledgements

This work was supported by grants from the Deutsche Forschungsgemeinschaft (Lu 443/1-3, So 87/11E).

References

1. Luger TA, Schwarz T. Effects of UV-light on cytokines and neuroendocrine hormones. In: *Photoimmunology*. Krutmann J, Elmets C (eds). Blackwell, Oxford, 1995: 55.
2. Scholzen T, Armstrong C, Luger TA, Ansel JC. Neuropeptides in the skin: interactions between the neuroendocrine and the skin immune system. *Exp Dermatol* 1998; 7 (in press).
3. Luger TA, Scholzen T, Grabbe S. The role of α-melanocyte stimulating hormone in cutaneous biology. *J Invest Dermatol, Derm Symp Proc* 1997; 2: 87.
4. Cone RD, Lu D, Koppula S, Vage DI, Klungland H, Boston B, Chen W, Orth DN, Pouton C, Kerterson RA. The melanocortin receptors: agonists, antagonists, and the hormonal control of pigmentation. *Recent Prog Horm Res* 1996; 51: 287.
5. Slominski A, Paus R, Wortsman J. On the potential role of proopiomelanocortin in skin physiology and pathology. *Mol Cell Endocrinol* 1993; 93: C1.
6. Luger TA, Beissert S, Schwarz T. The epidermal cytokine network. In: *Skin Immune System (SIS)*. J.D. Bos, ed., CRC Press, Boca Raton, 1997: 271.
7. Köck A, Schauer E, Schwarz T, Luger TA. Human keratinocytes synthesize and release neuropeptides such as α-MSH and ACTH. In: *Cellular and Cytokine Network in Tissue Immunity*. Meltzer M, Mantovani A, eds. John Wiley & Sons, Inc. New York, 1991: 105.
8. Brzoska T, Scholzen T, Becher E, Hartmeyer M, Bletz T, Schwarz T, Luger TA. UVB irradiation regulates the expression of proopiomelanocortin, prohormone convertase 1 and melanocortin receptor 1 by human keratinocytes. *J Invest Dermatol* 1997; 108: 622.
9. Bhardwaj RS, Becher E, Mahnke K, Hartmeyer M, Scholzen T, Schwarz T, Luger TA. Evidence of the expression of a functional melanocortin receptor 1 by human keratinocytes. *J Invest Dermatol* 1996; 106: 817.
10. Orel L, Simon MM, Karlseder J, Bhardwaj RS, Trautinger F, Schwarz T, Luger TA. Alpha-melanocyte stimulating hormone downregulates differentiation driven heat shock protein 70 expression in keratinocytes. *J Invest Dermatol* 1997; 108: 401.
11. Lipton JM, Catania A. Antiinflammatory actions of the neuroimmunomudulator α-MSH. Immunol Today 1997; 18: 140.
12. Bhardwaj RS, Schwarz A, Becher E, Mahnke K, Riemann H, Aragane Y. Pro-opiomelanocortin-derived petides induce IL-10 production in human monocytes. *J Immunol* 1996; 156: 2517.
13. Schwarz A, Grabbe S, Rieman H, Aragane Y, Simon M, Manon S, Andrade S, Luger TA, Zlotnik A, Schwarz T. In vivo effects of interleukin-10 on contact hypersensitivity and delayed-type hypersensitivity reactions. *J Invest Dermatol* 1994; 103: 211.

14. Grabbe S, Bhardwaj RS, Steinert M, Mahnke K, Simon MM, Schwarz T, Luger TA. Alpha-melanocyte stimulating hormone induces hapten-specific tolerance in mice. *J Immunol* 1996; 156: 473.
15. Bhardwaj RS, Becher E, Mahnke K, Hartmeyer M, Schwarz T, Scholzen T, Luger TA. Evidence for the differential expression of the functional alpha melanocyte stimulating hormone receptor MC-1 on human monocytes. *J Immunol* 1997; 158: 3378.
16. Star RA, Rajora N, Huang J, Chavez R, Catania A, Lipton JM. Evidence of autocrine modulation of macrophage nitric oxide synthase by alpha-MSH. *Proc Natl Acad Sci USA* 1995; 92: 8016.
17. Hartmeyer M, Scholzen T, Becher E, Bhardwaj RS, Fastrich M, Schwarz T, Luger TA. Human microvascular endothelial cells (HMEC-1) express the melanocortin receptor type 1 and produce increased levels of IL-8 stimulation with αMSH. *J Immunol* 1997; 159: 1930.
18. Kalden DH, Fastrich M, Brzoska T, Scholzen T, Hartmeyer M, Schwarz T, Luger TA. Alpha-melanocyte-stimulating hormone reduces endotoxin-induced activation of nuclear factor-κB in endothelial cells. *J Invest Dermatol* 1998; 110 (in press).

Relevance of photo-immunosuppression for viral infections (*i.e.* human papillomavirus)

B.J. Vermeer, J.N. Bouwes Bavinck

B.J. Vermeer, J.N. Bouwes Bavinck: Department of Dermatology, Leiden University Medical Center, PO Box 9600, 2300 RC Leiden, The Netherlands.

The relevance of photo-immunosuppression for human health is difficult to establish. Nevertheless, in animal models it has been shown that photo-immunosuppression can lead to a decreased immunoresponse against tumour-specific antigens [1] and infectious agents.

UVB exposure of rats before epicutaneous infection with the *Herpes simplex* virus led to a decreased cellular immune response [2]. It is recognized that UVB irradiation can suppress the immunological resistance to skin infections in mice [3, 4] as well as the resistance to non-skin associated infections [5]. When rabbits orally infected with *Trichinella* were exposed to UVB, these rabbits suffered from a severe infection with *Trichinella* [6].

In humans it is known that *Herpes simplex* virus infections are exacerbated by UV-exposure [7]. Apart from immunosuppression it has been shown that virus (*i.e.* HIV) can be activated by exposure to UVB-light [8]. Based on these data, we questioned whether human papillomavirus (HPV) infections, which are known to be the causative agents of warts, may also be exacerbated by UVB irradiation in humans. This question was especially relevant as we have shown that in renal transplant recipients the incidence of skin cancer increased considerably after transplantation [9]. The occurrence of skin cancer in these patients was predominantly present on sun-exposed areas of the skin. More precise data on the role of UV-light as an etiological agent in the development of skin cancer in these patients showed that the exposure to UV-light, received during childhood, played an additional role in the development of skin cancer [9].

The possible influence of exposure to UV-light on the development of skin cancer is shown in *Figure 1*. In this figure, we postulate that chronic exposure can lead to multiple mutations and that "acute" exposure may augment development of skin cancer via photo-immunosuppression.

Not only is the development of skin cancer, especially squamous cell carcinoma, prominent in transplant patients, these patients also develop wart-like lesions which resemble the lesions which are present in patients with the rare genetic syndrome called epidermodysplasia verricuformis (EV). In the wart-like lesions and the squamous cell carcinomas of these patients, DNA of EV-HPV can be detected. With the use of a nested PCR we were able to demonstrate the presence of EV-HPV-DNA in the squamous cell carcinomas of renal transplant recipients [10]. Also in about 50% of the wart-like lesions in transplant patients EV-HPV-DNA could be shown. An obvious question is whether the EV-HPVs are also present in the non-immunosuppressed population. We did not find EV-HPV-DNA in normal skin.

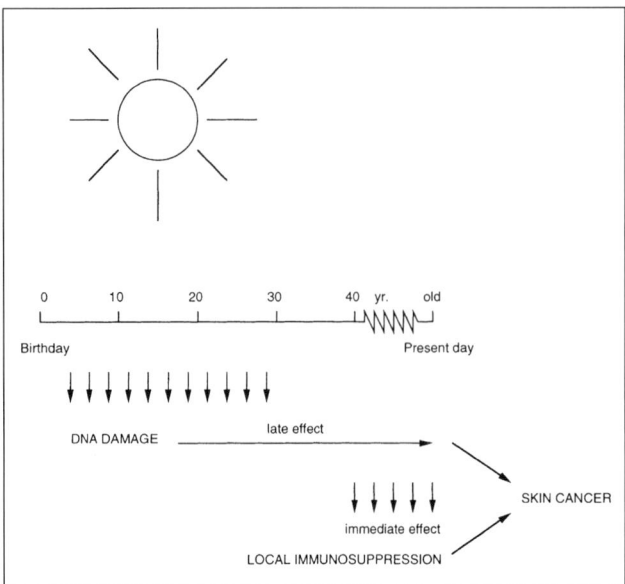

Figure 1. *Solar irradiation leads to DNA damage and multiple mutations. Local immunosuppression is induced as an immediate effect.*

However, in 40-80% of the squamous cell carcinomas and solar keratoses of non-immunosuppressed individuals EV-HPV-DNA could be detected.

Further research demonstrated that hair follicles may be the reservoir for these EV-HPVs. We found EV-HPV in plucked hairs in more than 40% of the normal population [11].

To further prove the hypothesis that HPV infections are associated with the development of skin cancer, we performed additional studies to investigate the immunological response against HPV antigens. An association between the production of antibodies against the L1-capsid antigen of HPV-8 and the occurrence of squamous cell carcinoma in renal transplant recipients was observed [12].

In the latter study, renal transplant recipients with squamous cell carcinoma had a lower prevalence of IgG antibodies against the HPV-8 L1 antigen. It was speculated that patients who had a deficient immune response against HPV-8 L1 consisting of an absent class switch from IgM to IgG antibodies may have an increased risk for the development of squamous cell carcinoma.

Recent studies in close collaboration with H. Pfister in Cologne, were focused on the detection of HPV-8 L1 antibodies by VLP-ELISA in the normal population and in a population who had solar keratoses and squamous cell carcinomas. The prevalence of antibodies against HPV-8 L1 in a normal population in Germany was 7%. However, in patients suffering from psoriasis who received PUVA treatment, 40% had antibodies against HPV-8 L1. In sero-epidemiological studies of the population of Saba, a small island in the Caribbean, we could demonstrate that the prevalence of HPV-8 L1 antibodies was significantly higher in patients with multiple solar keratoses and also in patients suffering from squamous cell carcinoma. Taken together, these serological data suggest that the immune response against HPV may play a role in the development of solar keratoses and squamous cell carcinoma. We formulate the hypothesis that photo-immunosuppression may decrease the immune response against HPV particles and in this way may play a role in the development of solar keratoses and squamous cell carcinoma. In non-immunosuppressed individuals the overall immune-response might be effective to such an extent, that the photo-immunosuppression has only an additional role. The effect of photo-immunosuppression may depend on genetic variations between individuals. This variation could be dependent on the HLA class I and class II phenotypes. These immune response genes determine the efficacy of the immune response against specific antigens, *i.e.* HPV. In view of this hypothesis it would be interesting to know whether sunscreens may prevent photo-immunosuppression. Regarding this subject, conflicting data have been forthcoming. However, clinical endpoint should be redefined. For instance since it has been shown that sunscreens can prevent the development of *Herpes simplex* virus infections, this could mean that photo-immunosuppression by UV-light could be prevented by that sunscreen. This clinical finding may be more relevant than many *in vitro* studies which are performed at the moment and which give many conflicting data. Along this line of thinking, the presence of EV-HPV infection in the skin may provide important data with which to assess the preventive effect of sunscreens on the development of solar keratosis and squamous cell carcinoma.

References

1. Kripke ML. Review. Effects of UV radiation on tumor immunity. *J Natl Cancer Inst* 1990; 82: 1392-5.
2. Goettsch W, Garssen J, Norval M, de Klerk A, van der Vliet H, Wildenbeest G, Dormans JAMA, El-Ghorr A, de Gruijl FR, van Loveren H. Effects of UVB exposure on the resistance to a skin-associated (HSV-1) and a non-skin associated (RCMV) Herpes infection in the rat. *Toxicol Lett* 1994; 72: 359-63.
3. Giannini MSH. Suppression of pathogenesis in cutaneous leishmanias by UV-radiation. *Infect Immunol* 1986; 51: 838-46.
4. Denkins YM, Fidler IJ, Kripke ML. Exposure of mice to UVB-radiation suppresses delayed hypersensitivity to Candida albicans. *Photochem Photobiol* 1989; 49: 615-9.
5. Jeevan A, Kripke ML. Alteration of immune responses to mycobacterium bovis BCG in mice exposed chronically to low doses of UV radiation. *Cell Immunol* 1989; 145: 2087-91.
6. Goettsch W, Garssen J, de Gruijl FR, van Loveren H. UVB exposure impairs resistance to infection with Trichinella spiralis. *Environm Health Perspect* 1994; 102: 298-301.
7. Norval M, El-Ghorr A, Garssen J, van Loveren H. The effect of ultraviolet light irradiation on viral infections. *Br J Dermatol* 1994; 130: 693-700.
8. Zmudzka BZ, Beer JZ, Yearly review. Activation of human immunodeficiency virus by ultraviolet radiation. *Photochem Photobiol* 1990; 52: 1153-62.
9. Bouwes Bavinck JN, de Boer A, Vermeer BJ, Hartevelt MM, van der Woude FJ, Claas FHJ, Wolterbeek R, Vandenbroucke JP. Sunlight, keratotic skin lesions and skin cancer in renal transplant recipients. *Br J Dermatol* 1993; 129: 242-9.
10. De Jong-Tieben LM, Berkhout RJM, Smits HL, Bouwes Bavinck JN, Vermeer BJ, van der Woude FJ, ter Schegget J. High frequency of detection of epidermodysplasia verruciformis associated human papillomavirus DNA in biopsies from malignant and premalignant skin lesions from renal transplant recipients. *J Invest Dermatol* 1995; 105: 367-71.
11. Boxman ILA, Berkhout RJM, Mulder LHC, Wolkers RC, Bouwes Bavinck JN, Vermeer BJ, ter Schegget J. Detection of human papilloma virus DNA in plucked hairs from renal transplant recipients and healthy volunteers. *J Invest Dermatol* 1997; 108: 712-5.
12. Bouwes Bavinck JN, Glissman L, Claas FHJ, van der Woude FJ, Persijn GG, ter Schegget J, Vermeer BJ, Jochmus I, Muller M, Steger G, Gebert S, Pfister H. Relation between skin cancer, humoral responses to human papillomaviruses and HLA class II molecules in renal transplant recipients. *J Immunol* 1993; 151: 1579-86.

Immunomodulation induced by psoralen plus ultraviolet A radiation

F. Aubin, Ph. Humbert

F. Aubin, Ph. Humbert: Department of Dermatology, University Hospital, Besançon, France.

Since 1974, psoralen plus ultraviolet A radiation (PUVA) has been widely used for the treatment of a variety of skin diseases. Because the pathology of diseases such as psoriasis, vitiligo, alopecia, lichen planus, atopic dermatitis, and graft-versus-host disease is thought to involve immune mechanisms, it has been suggested that at least some of the beneficial effects of PUVA may be due to its immunomodulatory properties. This paper reviews the mechanisms involved in the generation of immunosuppression during PUVA therapy.

Mice studies

Although both local and systemic PUVA treatment have been shown to cause immunosuppression [1, 2], the mechanisms underlying the induction of suppression are still not entirely clear. Studies in animals have demonstrated that dendritic epidermal cells are reduced in number and are morphologically altered following PUVA treatment [3, 4]. Treatment of mice with psoralen plus UVA radiation results in a striking reduction in the numbers of ATPase$^+$, Ia$^+$ dendritic epidermal cells. After 4 weeks of treatment (mice were treated 3 times per week with topical psoralen followed by 10 kJ/m^2 of UVA), the number of ATPase$^+$ cells was reduced by about 80% of control values [5]. The remaining positive cells exhibited morphologic alterations, including heavily stained, rounded cells with shortened dendrites. These results were observed regardless of whether the psoralen formed monofunctional or bifunctional adducts with DNA and regardless of its phototoxicity, except for 5-geranoxypsoralen which did not cause morphological alterations [6]. The reduction in the number of detectable cutaneous immune cells was accompanied by an impairment in the antigen-presenting activity of draining lymph node cell [5]. Draining lymph nodes cells from untreated mice sensitized with DNFB induced CHS when injected into the footpad of normal recipients. This antigen-presenting activity was markedly reduced in mice treated with PUVA therapy before sensitization. Because the suppression was reversed by cyclophosphamide treatment, Horio and Okamoto [1] suggested that suppressor cells may be involved. Different studies have confirmed that splenic suppressor cells are induced after local or systemic PUVA treatment [2, 5, 7]. Suppression of the CHS response was associated with the presence of suppressor lymphoid cells in the spleen of unresponsive mice, which transferred suppression to normal recipients. Okamoto et al. [8] have demonstrated that *in vivo* treatment of mice with PUVA diminished the ability of their spleen cells to produce IL-2 in culture. This impaired IL-2 production was not restored by adding IL-1 to the culture. This result indicates that the impairment was due to a primary defect in a population of a IL-2-producing cells rather than to a dysfunction of macrophages in the spleen. In addition, suppression of CHS and delayed type hypersensitivity (DTH) was transferred to normal recipients by soluble factors released from PUVA-treated keratinocytes. PAM 212 keratinocytes treated with psoralen plus high doses of UVA induced the release of a factor that depressed DTH to alloantigen. On the other hand, keratinocytes treated with psoralen plus lower doses of UVA released a factor that inhibited contact but not DTH response [9]. These results suggested that more than one immunosuppressive factors are involved in immunosuppression after PUVA treatment. The finding that both monofunctional and bifunctional psoralens can produce suppressive activity demonstrates that the formation of DNA cross-links is not required for induction of immunosuppression. This is not surprising because suppressor factors are released in response to UVA and UVB radiation alone [10, 11]. Beside the role of soluble mediators, expression of adhesion or co-stimulatory molecules by LC are required for activation of T cells. Exposure of Langerhans cells to PUVA completely inhibited their function and prevented increased expression of intercellular adhesion molecule-1 by LC *in vitro* [12].

Human studies

PUVA therapy reduces CHS to contact sensitizer applied through irradiated skin in humans [13, 14]. The immunosuppression induced by PUVA has been attributed mainly to the disappearance of epidermal LC [15] and decreases in their antigen-presenting capacity [16]. In addition, variable decreases in the numbers of the different subsets of circulating T-cells [17], particularly T helper cells [18] have been demonstrated. Kozeniztky *et al.* [19] demonstrated that PUVA has an inhibitory effect on cell proliferation, IL-2 production, and functional activity of T helper cells. Furthermore, a decrease in mRNA encoding for proinflammatory cytokines IL-6, IL-8, and TNF-a has been observed both *in vitro* and *in vivo*, in PUVA-treated peripheral blood mononuclear cells from healthy individuals [20]. More recently, we found that the percentage of $CD3^+$ peripheral lymphocytes producing IFN-g and IL-2 was reduced during PUVA therapy in patients with psoriasis [21]. Our data support the hypothesis of an anergy of type 1 activity in peripheral lymphocytes induced by photochemotherapy as suggested by in vivo UVB-irradiated mouse models [22].

Mechanisms of PUVA-induced immune suppression

While the photobiological effect of PUVA therapy is beginning to be well known, the mechanisms of PUVA-induced immune suppression are not completely understood : induction of monofunctional and/or bifunctional adducts within DNA [23], interactions with specific receptor [24], photo-isomerization of urocanic acid [25], free-radical formation [26, 27], and signal transduction-mediated activation of transcription factors [28] may play a role. Indeed, plasma-membrane changes and the concomitant cytoplasmic alterations and nuclear alterations have been demonstrated in different cell lines treated by PUVA [26, 29]. However, there remain a number of important additional issues that must be resolved. What is the biochemical composition of the various suppressive substances? How do these factors induce suppressor cells? What is the primary photoreceptor? In conclusion, these data suggest that PUVA therapy-induced immune suppression is likely to be involved in the therapeutic effect observed in T cell mediated skin condition.

References

1. Horio T, Okamoto H. The mechanisms of inhibitory effect of 8-methoxypsoralen and longwave ultraviolet light on experimental contact sensitization. *J Invest Dermatol* 1982; 78: 402-5.
2. Kripke ML, Morison WL, Parrish JA. Systemic suppression of contact hypersensitivity in mice by psoralen plus UVA radiation. *J Invest Dermatol* 1983; 81: 87-92.
3. Aberer W, Schuler G, Stingl G, Hönigsmann H, Wolff K. Ultraviolet light depletes surface markers on Langerhans cells. *J Invest Dermatol* 1981; 76: 781-94.
4. Koulu L, Christer T, Jansen CT, Viander M. Effect of UVA and UVB irradiation on human epidermal Langerhans cell membrane markers defined by ATPase activity and monoclonal antibodies (OKT 6 and anti-Ia). *Photodermatology* 1985; 2: 339-46.
5. Aubin F, Dall'acqua F, Kripke ML. Local suppression of contact hypersensitivity in mice by a new bifunctional psoralen, 4,4'5'-trimethylazapsoralen, plus UVA radiation. *J Invest Dermatol* 1991; 95: 50-4.
6. Aubin F, Humbert Ph, Agache P. Effects of a new psoralen, 5-geranoxypsoralen, plus UVA radiation on murine ATPase positive Langerhans cells. *J Dermatol Sci* 1994; 7: 176-84.
7. Alcaaly J, Ullrich SE, Kripke ML. Local suppression of contact hypersensitivity in mice by a monofunctional psoralen plus UVA radiation. *Photochem Photobiol* 1989; 50: 217-20.
8. Okamoto H, Horio T, Maeda M. Alteration of lymphocyte function by 8-methoxypsoralen and long-wave ultraviolet radiation. II: the effect of in vivo PUVA on IL-2 production. *J Invest Dermatol* 1987; 89: 24-6.
9. Aubin F, Ullrich SE, Kripke ML. Activation of keratinocytes with psoralen plus UVA radiation induces the release of soluble factors that suppress delayed and contact hypersensitivity. *J Invest Dermatol* 1991; 97: 995-1000.
10. Kim TY, Kripke ML, Ullrich SE. Immunosuppression by factors released from UV-irradiated epidermal cells: selective effects on the generation of contact and delayed hypersensitivity after exposure to UVA or UVB radiation. *J Invest Dermatol* 1990; 94: 26-32.
11. Ullrich SE, McIntyre BW, Rivas JM. Suppression of the immune response to alloantigen by factors released from ultraviolet-irradiation keratinocytes. *J Immunol* 1990; 145: 489-98
12. Tang A, Udey MC. Doses of ultraviolet radiation that modulate accessory cell activity and ICAM-1 expression are ultimately cytotoxic for murine epidermal Langerhans cells. *J Invest Dermatol* 1992; 99: 71S-73S.
13. Strauss GH, Greaves M, Price M, Bridges BA, Hall-Smith P, Vella-Biffa. Inhibition of delayed hypersensitivity reaction in skin (DNCB test) by 8-methoxypsoralen photochemotherapy. *Lancet* 1980; 2: 556-9.
14. Moss C, Friedmann PS, Shuster S. Impaired contact hypersensitivity in untreated psoriasis and the effects of photochemotherapy and dithranol/UVB. *Br J Dermatol* 1981; 105: 503-8.
15. Koulu L, Soderstrom KO, Jansen CT. Relation of antipsoriatic and Langerhans cell depleting effects of systemic psoralen photochemotherapy: a clinical, enzyme histochemical, and electron microscopic study. *J Invest Dermatol* 1984; 82: 591-3.
16. Ashwoth J, Kahan MC, Breathnach. PUVA therapy decreases HLA-DR+, CD1a+ Langerhans cells and epidermal cell antigen-presenting capacity in human skin, but flow cytometrically-sorted residual HLA-DR$^+$ CD1a$^+$ Langerhans cells exhibit normal alloantigen-presenting function. *Br J Dermatol* 1989; 120: 329-39.
17. Moscicki RA, Morison WL, Parrish JA, Bloch KJ, Colvin RB. Reduction of the fraction of circulating helper-inducer T-cells identified by monoclonal antibodies in psoriatic patients treated with long-term psoralen/ultraviolet-A radiation (PUVA). *J Invest Dermatol* 1982; 79: 205-8.
18. Borroni G, Zaccone C, Vignati G, Fietta A, Gatti M, Brazelli V, Rabbiosi G. Lymphopenia and decrease in the total number of circulating CD3$^+$ and CD4$^+$ T-cells during long-term PUVA treatment for psoriasis. *Dermatologica* 1991; 183: 10-4.
19. Kozenitzky L, David M, Sredni B, Albeck M, Shohat B. Immunomodulatory effects of AS101 on interleukin-2 production and T-lymphocyte function of lymphocytes treated with psoralens and ultraviolet A. *Photodermatol Photoimmunol Photomed* 1992; 9: 24-8.

20. Neuner P, Charvat B, Knobler R, Kirnbauer R, Schwarz A, Luger T, Schwarz T. Cytokine release by peripheral blood mononuclear cells is affected by 8-methoxypsoralen plus UVA. *Photochem Photobiol* 1994; 59: 182-8.
21. Aubin F, Dufour MP, Billot M, Racadot E, Humbert Ph. Effects of treatment with psoralen plus ultraviolet A radiation on the production of cytokines Th1 and Th2 by peripheral lymphocytes in patients with psoriasis (submitted).
22. Ullrich SE. Does exposure to UV radiation induce a shift to a Th2-like immune reaction? *Photochem Photobiol* 1996; 64: 254-8.
23. Pathak MA. Mechanisms of psoralen photosensitization reactions. *Natl Cancer Inst Monograph* 1984; 66: 41-6.
24. Laskin JD, Lee E, Yurkow EJ, Laskin DL, Gallo MA. A possible mechanism of psoralen phototoxicity not involving direct interaction with DNA. *Proc Natl Acad Sci USA* 1985; 82: 6158-62.
25. Norval M, Gibbs NK, Gilmour J. The role of urocanic acid in UV-induced immunosuppression: recent advances (1992-1994). *Photochem Photobiol* 1995; 62: 209-17.
26. Malinin GI, Lo HK, Hornicek FJ, Malinin TI. Ultrastructural modification of the plasma membrane in HUT 102 lymphoblasts by long-wave ultraviolet light, psoralen, and PUVA. *J Invest Dermatol* 1990; 95: 97-103.
27. Punnonen K, Jansen CT, Puntal A, Ahotupa M. Effects of in vitro irradiation and PUVA treatment on membrane fatty acids and activities of antioxydant enzymes in human keratinocytes. *J Invest Dermatol* 1991; 96: 255-9.
28. Tokura Y, Edelson RL, Gasparro FP. Modulation of 8-methoxypsoralen-DNA-photoadduct formation by cell differentiation, mitogenic stimulation and phorbol ester exposure in murine T-lymphocytes. *Photochem Photobiol* 1993; 58: 822-6.
29. Ree K, Johnsen AS, Hovig T. Ultrastructural studies on the effects of photoactivated 8-methoxy psoralen. *Acta Path Microbiol Scand Sect A* 1981; 89: 81-90.

Recent advances in sun protection

H. Schaefer, D. Moyal, A. Fourtanier

H. Schaefer, D. Moyal, A. Fourtanier: L'Oréal Research, Clichy, France.

The prevention of photodermatoses implies that the exposure of photosensitive patients to UV light is reduced to levels below the threshold of induction of light reactions. The four principal measures of prevention are the following:
- avoidance of sun exposure around noontime,
- UV-protective clothes,
- hats,
- use of sunscreen products.

Protection of photosensitive patients by sunscreen products plays an important role. This is particularly true for the prevention of photodermatoses which are elicited by UV-A. About 50% of the exposure to UV-A occurs in the shade, *i.e.* in the absence of direct sunlight. The amount of UV-A in sunlight is high from sunrise to sunset, whereas the intensity of UV-B peaks more sharply at noontime. Whereas window and car glass materials offer an effective shield against UV-B, they are transparent for UV-A.

Moreover, due to the presence of subclinical and/or apparent eczema in already affected skin areas, the natural protective capacity of the horny layer may be reduced or lost altogether, which will further increase the light sensitivity of the afflicted skin.

Which are the ideal properties of state-of-the-art sun protection products?
Such compounds should be:
i. well tolerated
ii. cosmetically pleasant
iii. non-toxic
iv. equally effective against UV-A and UV-B
v. photostable
vi. wateresistant
vii. with a high "Sun Protection Factor"

These criteria should be briefly commented (adverse properties listed under i., through iii. are exclusion criteria).

i. Good tolerance is of primary importance, since such products are often applied to sensitive skin and under stress conditions. Skin tolerance requires careful testing and optimisation, since preparations with high protection factors contain relatively large amounts of UV filter substances (see below). Many promising filter substances are rejected at an early stage of development due to their irritant, photoirritant or photoallergic potential.

ii. Patient compliance depends above all on the easy and agreeable use of the sunscreen. In other words: the product should be invisible and should not have unpleasant cosmetic properties (not whitish/greasy/glossy/sticky). In addition, the substance should be colourless and tasteless.

iii. Sun protection products are applied to a large body surface. This means that percutaneous absorption of filter substances (which, except for water insoluble inorganic substances such as titanium dioxide, is never zero) must not produce adverse effects. The safety of filter substances is determined by comparison of the so-called "No Adverse Effect Level" (NOAEL) to the potential human exposure. The NOAEL is determined by subchronic (90 to 180 days) or chronic (> 180 days) (mostly oral) toxicity studies in a test animal population, generally in rats. Such studies are performed with the objective to define a safe dose of the substance and generally use several dose levels. The daily dose at which no toxic effect can be observed is called the NOAEL. In other words, the NOAEL is a daily dose which can be tolerated by the organism for a considerable period of time without producing measurable toxicity. The NOAEL is expressed in mg/kg body weight per day. After the NOAEL has been established, the percutaneous absorption of the substance will be quantified and calculated in mg/kg body weight. Only such filter substances are acceptable which have a large "margin of safety" (MoS), *i.e.* the relation of the potentially penetrated dose compared to the NOAEL, are accepted as safe. The MoS should at least be 100x. When comparing the toxicological properties of known UV-B and UV-A filters to the potential human exposure, the human risk due to systemic exposure to filter substances is very low and may be ignored altogether. (Dermatologist should keep in mind that, comparatively, the potential systemic damage by UV light, in particular by the deeply penetrating UV-A to blood cells passing through the skin microvasculature is not to be neglected). Furthermore, state-of-the-art preparations of modern UV filters are formulated to be retained on or within the upper layers of the horny layer, since such products achieve the highest protection factors.

iv. Of particular importance for the prevention of photodamage in general and photodermatoses in particular is the absorption spectrum of sun protection products. In the past, all sun protection products were assessed according to protocols which measured UV-induced erythema. In fact, the erythema is largely due to UV-B whereas exceedingly high doses of UV-A are needed to elicit an acute erythema response. However, only in recent years the more predominant role of UV-A in chronic photodamage and in acute and chronic photodermatoses has became apparent (see below). As to more recent concerns about the potential risk of photo-immune depression, it is far from clear, which immune mechanisms are affected by which part of the UV spectrum. Thus, although the damage to DNA and the respective risk of skin cancer formation may be predominantly due to UV-B, a complete protection requires the coverage of the entire UV spectrum. Therefore, the development of UV-A-absorbing filter substances became an important but difficult goal: the better a compound absorbs in long wave UV-A region (the spectrum close to visible light), the more the substance tends to be coloured (mostly yellow) and instable to UV-light. This explains why only few UV-A absorbers became commercially available. Today, state-of-the-art sun products are based on combinations of several filter substances, which result in a homogenous absorption spectrum over the full range of UV light. The development of suitable combinations and their formulation is a long – and admittedly empirical – process which yielded improved and broader protection while using with the same or lower concentrations of filter substances.

v. A protection is only as good as the stability of the protective product. This sounds obvious when it concerns the prevention of UV light-mediated skin disorders. However most photochemical processes, which occur when the energy of a photon hitting a UV absorbing substance is dissipated, are irreversible: the compound may undergo a photoreaction, may break apart or become otherwise inactivated; in other words, the filter may be consumed by the irradiation. The more photoinstable a filter substance, the more rapidly it is consumed under exposure. Only when the UV energy is quantitatively transformed into infrared radiation, *i.e.* into heat, the process is reversible: the respective filter or filter combination is photostable and provides protection for several hours. The best filter substances are photostable as such (*e.g.* Mexoryl® SX). However, they are not yet world-wide available. The problems of photoinstability may be overcome – within limits – by careful selection of combinations, whereby the substances stabilise each other mutually against photo-degradation. However, there is a caveat which is hardly ever evoked: consider that the stratum corneum sheds off one layer of squames per day, *i.e.* on the average one third of a layer in 8 hours. This shedding is irregular, some areas shed off larger scales other stay unchanged for a considerable period of time. The desquamation is accelerated under physical stress including UV exposure. Since the most efficient filters are those remaining on and in the upper layers of the horny layer, their efficiency is reduced by this process. Thus one should not expect – due to inherent aspects of skin physiology and pathophysiology – that the protection by the best possible product can last longer than a few hours before becoming patchy.

vi. Water resistance is another obvious criterion of quality. This property can only be achieved by a careful choice of vehicle ingredients, in particular when water-soluble filter substances are used. However, increased water solubility provides a higher affinity to the proteinous part of the stratum corneum. Nevertheless a clean skin surface is the best basis for efficient protection, since loose squames and decomposing skin surface lipids may easily be washed off by sweat or sea water and may thus remove the sunscreens.

vii. An important issue is the level of Sun Protection Factor (SPF). Recent findings suggest that high SPFs (> 15) are needed to ascertain an adequate protection. However, published guidelines suggest determination of the SPF should be performed with a solar simulator which generates UV light which contains an excess of erythemal UVB and an insufficient quantity of UVA. This UV light can not be compared to the actual solar light (the spectrum of the simulator corresponds to sunlight at noon time and at several thousands meters of altitude). With such a light source the SPFs are clearly overestimated [1, 2]. A second important point is that SPFs are determined using an applied amount of 2 mg/cm^2 of sunscreen whereas patients or consumers normally apply only between 0.5 and 1 mg/cm^2 of product. This reduces the in-use protection by a factor of more than 2-fold [3-5]. To achieve high SPFs, products must combine UVA and UVB absorbers. Therefore, in addition to indicating the SPF, a product should be tested for UVA protection and a respective factor should be listed on the label. However, methods for determination of UVA protection factors are still under discussion and no standard method has yet been accepted. The discussion on a harmonized standard protocol for the determination of UVA protection is ongoing and *in vitro* or *in vivo* assays have been proposed. As *in vitro* methods do not take into account interactions between the sunscreen product and the skin and the possible photoinstability of the product it seems recommendable to use an *in vivo* method. Erythema can be used but it is a rather impractical endpoint since its induction requires long exposure time and high UVA energy. Another possibility is to use the immediate (IPD) or the persistent pigment darkening reaction (PPD) observed immediately or 2 hours after UVA exposure. This reaction, which corresponds to a photooxydation of melanin, occurs in the horny layer of all skin types except skin type I. PPD is preferable over IPD because the pigmentation remains stable between 2 and 24 hours [6].

UV-induced cell damage and its prevention by sunscreens

DNA damage

There is general agreement that DNA is one of the main targets of UV-induced skin damage leading to a variety of adverse effects such as immunosuppression, sunburn cell formation, mutation and, ultimately, carcinogenesis. Within the DNA the pyrimidine bases are more sensitive to UV. These bases undergo a number of modifications due to direct absorption of photons or free radicals generated by the absorption of photons by chromophores. The major molecular lesions are cyclobutane dimers and pyrimidine [4, 6] pyrimidone photoproducts [7, 8]. Normally these lesions are repaired. However, if the enzymes are not functional or if the repair system is overloaded, mutations appear in the DNA [9].

As both UVB and UVA induce DNA lesions [9], it is important that the absorption spectrum of sunscreens should be as broad as possible. Recent studies have shown that such sunscreens are able to prevent DNA damage and their consequences.

For example, two UV absorbers have been reported to prevent the induction of pyrimidine dimers in the DNA of cutaneous cells: a UVB absorber (2-ethyl-hexyl-p-methoxycinnamate, 2-EHMC, Parsol® MCX), and a broad spectrum UVA filter (terephtalylidene dicamphor sulfonic acid, TDSA, Mexoryl SX). This protective effect has been observed in a study in mice [10] and in a study in humans, respectively [11]. Both absorbers were evaluated at 5% (w/w) in a similar vehicle, and the SPF of the 2 preparations were equal to 4.

In the study in humans the DNA protection factor was found comparable to the SPF, indicating that protection from erythema by a UVB or a broad spectrum UVA sunscreen results in a proportional protection against DNA photolesions. In the mouse, both UV filters offered a greater protection of DNA than predicted by their SPF, although the efficacy of TDSA was superior than that of 2-EHMC.

Skin cancer

There are numerous animal studies showing that sunscreens are effective in preventing skin cancer development. Only few of them are using a correct UV source (*i.e.* a solar simulator). In a recent one the efficacy of the two previously cited UV filters was evaluated [12]. It was demonstrated that both the broad spectrum UVA filter TDSA and the UVB filter 2-EHMC delayed significantly the tumor development. An unexpected result was found: TDSA, the broad UVA spectrum absorber, delayed tumor appearance significantly longer than 2-EHMC. Neither the SPF values (4 for both products), nor the currently available photocarcinogenesis action spectra [13] would have predicted this outcome. These results confirm that a broad filtration is superior to narrow one, particularly for protection against DNA damage and photocarcinogenesis. These data suggest that sunscreens prevent development of carcinomas. Furthermore these results also suggest that, for prevention of skin cancer, protection against UVA may be as important as protection against UVB Two recent studies in humans, one in the US and one in Australia, demonstrated that repeated sunscreen applications may reduce the development of actinic keratoses, which are considered to be precancerous lesions [14, 15].

Mutations

UV radiation induces mutations in important genes. One gene has been extensively studied during the recent years, the P 53 tumor suppressor gene, the "guardian of the genome". It has been shown that more than 80% of sun-induced human skin cancers contain P 53 mutations at dipyrimidine sites [16] suggesting that this gene plays an important role in the development of UV-induced skin tumours. In a recent publication Ananthaswamy *et al.* [17] reported that such mutations can be detected in UV-irradiated mouse skin months before the appearance of tumours and that application of sunscreens prevented the appearance of these mutations.

Immunosuppression

Ultraviolet radiation has been shown to induce immunosuppression. This phenomenon plays an important role in UV carcinogenesis by contributing to a decrease of the host resistance against tumor growth [18]. UV alters antigen presenting cell function by affecting directly the number, the morphology and functionality of Langerhans cells [19, 20]. It induces also the release of immunomodulating cytokines [21] and the isomerisation of urocanic acid (UCA) from trans- to cis form. The cis isomer of UCA has been reported to play an important role in the initiation of photoimmunosuppression [22, 23].

All these effects are induced by UVB and UVA and may impair the induction of local and systemic contact hypersensitivity (CHS) and delayed type reactions (DTH) to hapten applied to irradiated or unirradiated skin [24-30]. The precise mechanisms by which UV radiation induces immune suppression are still unclear.

Contradictory results have been reported on the potential of sunscreens to protect against this phenomenon [31-36].

Dermatoheliosis or photoaging

There is compelling evidence to support that UVB in sunlight induces photoaging [39, 40]. More recent studies on animals and humans [41-44] suggest that UVA also contributes to the changes observed in photo-damaged skin.

The changes produced in normal human skin by repeated daily exposures to low doses of UVA and to simulated solar radiation and the prevention offered by sunscreens were recently studied in our laboratory.

In the first study, the efficacy of Mexoryl® SX a broad UVA absorber (λ max = 345 nm) against the UVA induced changes in human skin was examined [45]. The regimen of UVA exposure (13 weeks with increasing suberythemal doses) induced a strong pigmentation but no erythema. Skin hydration and elasticity decreased whereas the total skin thickness, assessed by echography, as well as epidermal thickness, histologically measured, remained unchanged. However irradiated epidermis had a thickened stratum corneum and an increase in the expression of ferritin an iron storage protein. No significant alterations were measured using antisera against type IV collagen or laminin suggesting that the dermal epidermal junction (DEJ) was preserved. In the dermis, enhanced expression of tenascin was measured just below the DEJ but type I procollagen which is localized at the same site was unaltered. Although we were unable to visualize any change in the elastic network organization using Luna staining or specific antiserum against human elastin, we noticed an increased deposition of lysozyme or alpha 1-antitrypsin on elastin fibers. All changes noticed in the irradiated group were not observed in the group treated with the UVA filter. Therefore, a broad UVA filter (5%) efficiently prevents UV induced alterations.

Because exposure to pure UVA is not a normal occurrence, the changes induced by exposure to repeated full-spectrum UV (solar simulated radiation = SSR) were examined [46]. The preventive activity of a formulation containing UVB and UVA filters was evaluated. Minimal erythemal dose of SSR was applied 5 days per week for 6 weeks, with or without the sunscreen to unexposed buttock of 12 healthy caucasian volunteers. This regimen induced the following effects :

– melanogenesis,
– decrease in skin hydration and alterations of the skin microtopography associated with a thickening of the stratum corneum and the stratum granulosum,
– enhanced expression of tenascin and a decreased expression of the type I procollagen (UVB markers),
– increased deposition of lysozyme and alpha-1 antitrypsin (UVA markers) on elastin fibers, likely contributing to solar induced elastosis process.

The sunscreen combination cream prevented UVB and UVA induced alterations. These results demonstrate the efficacy of a photostable combination of UV filters covering the entire UV spectrum.

Photodermatoses

UV plays a role in the pathogenesis of various photodermatoses [47, 48]. Several drugs or substances may induce photosensitization (photoallergy or phototoxicity) when used topically or orally. The wavelengths which cause activation of most phototoxic drugs or photoallergens is in the UVA range. Idiopathic photodermatoses such as actinic prurigo and hydroa vacciniforme are mainly UVA-induced. UVA may play a important role in the pathogenesis of polymorphic light eruption or benign summer light eruption and in lupus erythematosus. Patients suffering from such disorders should use broad-spectrum sunscreens containing UVB as well as UVA filters. It has been shown that broad-spectrum sunscreens can efficiently protect patients against polymorphic light eruption [49], benign summer light eruption [50] and lupus erythematosus [51].

In our laboratory we studied particularly the prevention of Polymorphous Light Eruption (PLE). PLE is an idiopathic photodermatosis frequently found in humans originating from the Northern parts of Europe.

PLE generally occurs after at least two sufficiently intensive exposures to sunlight. The cutaneous lesions take various forms: generally, they consist of papules, reticulated erythema, vesicles and pruritus. They appear only on those areas which were exposed to sunlight. They are principally located on the chest, arms, abdomen and legs but in the most severe cases can spread further, affecting the face.

Although the light wavelengths incriminated in the triggering of PLE may include the entire ultraviolet (UV) spectrum it is commonly recognised that PLE is mainly caused by UVA. It is also possible that the use of certain sunscreens that mainly protect the skin against UVB cause an increase in the incidence of PLE [52].

Various treatments have been proposed to prevent the onset of PLE: Psoralen-UVA (PUVA) therapy and UVB phototherapy afford protection in 60-90% of cases.
Other forms of treatment, such as oral β-carotene or hydroxychloroquine had only limited success. Protection by the topical route with UVB filters or an insufficient level of protection against UVA has been ineffective.

We carried out different studies to reproduce PLE under simulated and actual sunlight to evaluate the efficacy of different sunscreen products to prevent the eruption. The studies were carried out in women of Caucasian origin, aged from 18 to 50 years, and phototype II to IV. All subjects reported to have suffered from PLE and were selected according to their medical history; antinuclear factors were negative. The subjects were included in the studies following a clinical examination and after informed consent. None of the subjects had been exposed to UV for at least 3 months.

In the first study we confirmed the role of UVA in the onset of PLE. The subjects were exposed solely on the chest, the predominant site of the PLE. A total of 52 subjects were included and exposed without photoprotection under a UVASUN metal halide lamp with an emission spectrum from 330 to 440 nm. The subjects were exposed in a single daily application for a total of max. 5 days from 25 J/cm^2 to 35 J/cm^2/day), the equivalent of about 1.5 hours sunshine at noon in Mediterraneen countries.

The clinical examination was performed approximately 5 hours after each exposure, as PLE is not immediately visible after the completion of exposure.

Objective signs such as erythema, papules and oedema, and subjective symptoms (burning and pruritus) were rated on a 4-point severity scale.

Outbreak of PLE was observed on 49/50 patients. In the majority of cases, outbreak was observed on the third day after a cumulated UVA dose of 80 J/cm^2.

In a second study we confirmed that UVB exacerbates PLE when combined with UVA.
Following these studies it appeared appropriate to use a sunlamp with a UVB/UVA spectrum for indoor studies of the preventive efficacy of sunscreen products.

The solar simulator used was a SUPERSUN Lamp with an emission spectrum from 290 to 390 nm.

A study was performed to evaluate the prevention of PLE by a UVA/UVB sunscreen which offers high UVA and UVB photoprotection and contains a photostable combination of Avobenzone (Parsol 1789), 4-methylbenzylidene-camphor (Eusolex 6300) terephtalylidene dicamphor sulfonic acid (Mexoryl® SX) together with micronised titanium dioxide.
For comparison a UVB-selective sunscreen was included.

The study was carried out over 5 consecutive days. Each morning the test substances (2 mg/cm^2) were applied to the right or left half of the chest in a randomised manner.
Each subjects' neckline was then exposed to the sunlamp. Each day, the UVB doses were increased progressively. The highest UV dose was equivalent to 2 hours exposure to the mid-

day sun. As described above, evaluation for PLE was performed approximately 5 hours after UV exposure.

On day three, 12/18 volunteers developed PLE on the side of the chest protected by UVB sunscreen.

No PLE was detected on the side protected by the UVB/UVA sunscreen.

On day four, all 18/18 subjects had developed PLE on the side protected by the UVB sunscreen.

On day five, only one subject had signs of PLE on the side protected by the UVB-UVA sunscreen.

The study confirm that PLE may be produced indoors, using a sunlamp with a UVA/UVB spectrum. This method appears more suitable than UVA irradiation alone, since PLE appeared at lower cumulative UVA doses (89 J/cm^2) as compared to the doses when UVA is used alone (145 J/cm^2). Under these conditions a sunscreen providing high level protection against UVA as well as UVB effectively prevents PLE.

Using the same protocol we compared the efficacy of two high SPF sunscreen products which had different efficacy in the UVA range: SPF 60 – UVA PF 12 and SPF 50 – UVA PF4.

The study was carried out on 14 female subjects who were susceptible to PLE.
After 5 days and a total UVA dose of 150 J/cm^2 we observed only two cases of slight PLE with the SPF 60 UVA PF12 sunscreen and 14 cases of PLE with the SPF 50 UVA PF 4 product. This confirmed that a high level of protection in the UVA range is essential for the prevention of PLE.

These studies were then complemented by an investigation under natural sunlight using realistic conditions of exposure.

The first study was conducted in Guadelupe (latitude 16°15N, longitude 15°35W) on 20 PLE-susceptible female subjects. A half-body site comparison was made between a commercial product type P1 that filters only in the UVB spectrum and, hence, protects from actinic erythema and a protectant of type P2 that possesses good UVB-filtering capacity and a UVA protection factor of 4.

Our results showed that after use of the sunscreen which protects only in the UVB range PLE appeared rapidly (90% at day 3). Use of the UVB/UVA filter prevented PLE in 6/20 subjects, whereas in the 14 remaining subjects the onset of PLE was delayed and its degree less severe.

Further studies were carried out under natural sunlight in Djerba, Tunisia (latitude 33°50N, longitude 10°48E), where the efficacy of products with higher UVA protection factor was compared. Thirty-five women were protected on half-body by a product containing solely UVB filters (P1) and on the other half by a product of class P3 (UVA PF between 6 and 9). Eight additional subjects whose susceptibility to PLE in the sun, when protected only by a P1 product, was well known served for an additional study to compare the efficacy of a product of class P3 with a UVA-PF between 6 and 9 with that of a product P4 with an UVA PF of > 10.

In 27/43 subjects who received a P3-type product a complete prevention of PLE was recorded. In the remaining subjects, the onset of their PLE was delayed and/or its severity reduced when compared to the effect of the UVB filter (type P1). In the 8 subjects who received a product of P4 type, PLE was not observed.

We conclude from these studies that UVA plays a dominant role in the induction of PLE. The findings demonstrate that state of the art sunscreen products prevent the onset of this PLE. Maximal prevention was achieved by sunscreen products providing a high protection throughout the entire UV spectrum and, in particular, the UVA spectrum. The best results were obtained by using a combination of two complementary UVA filters Avobenzone and Mexoryl® SX, which allow a high level of UVA absorbance and completely prevented PLE.

Conclusion

During recent years, novel and highly efficient sunscreens have been developed. Health authorities, dermatologists and the cosmetic industry should now educate their patients or consumers in the use (quantity, application) and the selection of a good sunscreen product. Commercial products should list their UVAPF. The UVAPF should be determined by standardized and relevant method. State-of-the-art sunscreens should be photostable, have a high SPF-Broad Spectrum and include UVA and UVB absorbers. Patients and consumers should be educated not to limit the use of sunscreens to outdoors or the summer months. Given that repeated minor exposure episodes account for 80% of the total lifetime exposure protection during these small periods is crucial. Thus the goal of sun protection should not be limited to protection against acute effects such as sunburn or photodermatoses, but should include prevention of long-term skin damage and reduction in the risk of skin cancer.

References

1. Uhlmann B, Mann T, Gers-Barlag H, Alert D, Sauermann G. Consequences for sun protection factors when solar simulator spectra deviate from the spectrum of the sun. *Int J Cosm Sc* 1996; 18: 13-24.
2. Sayre RM, Kollias N, Ley RD, Bager AH. Changing the risk spectrum of injury and the performance of sunscreen products throughout the day. *Photodermatol Photoimmunol Photomed* 1994; 10: 148-53.
3. Bech-Thomsen N, Wulf HC. Sunbather's application of sunscreen is probably inadequate to obtain the sun protection factor assigned to the preparation. *Photodermatol Photoimmunol Photomed* 1992,1993; 9: 242-4.
4. Toda K, Pathak MA. Determination of sun protection values of three test products under indoor and outdoor test conditions using Japanese volunteers. *J Jpn Cosmet Sci Soc* 1988; 12: 139-44.
5. Wulf HC, Stender IM, Lock-Andersen J. Sunscreens used at the beach do not protect against erythema: a new definition of SPF is proposed. *Photodermatol Photoimmunol Photomed* 1997; 13: 129-32.
6. Chardon A, Moyal D, Hourseau C. Persistent pigment darkening response as a method for evaluation of ultraviolet A protection assays. *In : Sunscreens, 2nd edition* (Edited by N.J. Lowe, Nadim A. Shaath, Madhu A. Pathak) Marcel Dekker, Inc. New-York, Basel, Hong-Kong 1997: 559-82.

7. Setlow RB. DNA damage and repair: A Photobiological Odyssey. *Photochem Photobiol* 1997; 655: 1195-225.
8. Bishop JM. Molecular themes in oncogenesis. *Cell* 1991; 64: 234-48.
9. Cadat J, Berger M, Douki T, Morin B, Raoul S, Ravanat JL, Spinelli S. Effects of UV and visible radiation on DNA final base damage. *Biol Chem* 1997; 378: 1275-86.
10. Ley RD, Fourtanier A. Sunscreen protection against ultraviolet radiation-induced pyrimidine dimers in mouse epidermal DNA. *Photochem Photobiol* 1997; 65: 1007-11.
11. Young AR, Sheehan JM, Chadwhick CA, Potten CS. Sunscreens afford protection against DNA photodamage in human epidermis *in situ*. *Photochem Photobiol* 1998; 67: 19S.
12. Fourtanier A. Mexoryl® SX protects against solar simulated UVR induced photocarcinogenesis in mice. *Photochem Photobiol* 1996; 64: 688-93.
13. De Gruijl FR, Sterenborg HJC, Forbes PD, Davies RE, Cole C, Kelfens G, Van Weelden H, Slaper H, Van Der Leun JC. Wavelength dependence of skin cancer induction by ultraviolet irradiation of albino hairless mice. *Cancer Res* 1993; 53: 53-60.
14. Thompson SC, Jolley D, Mark R. Reduction of solar keratoses by regular sunscreen use. *N Engl J Med* 1993; 329: 1147-51.
15. Naylor MF, Boyd A, Smith DW, *et al*. High sun protection factor (SPF) sunscreens in the suppression of active neoplasia. *Arch Dermatol* 1995; 131: 170-5.
16. Levine AJ, Momand J, Finland CA. The P53 mutations in human cancers. *Science* 1991; 253: 49-53.
17. Ananthaswamy HN, Loughlin SM, Cox P, Evans RL, Ullrich SE, Kripke ML. Sunlight and skin cancer: inhibition of P53 mutations in UV irradiated mouse skin by sunscreens. *Nature Med* 1997; 3: 510-4.
18. Nishigori C, Yarosh DB, Donawho C, *et al*. The immune system in ultraviolet carcinogenesis. *J Invest Dermatol Symp Proc* 1996: 143-6.
19. Ullrich SE. Modulation of immunity by ultraviolet radiation: key effects on antigen presentation. *J Invest Dermatol* 1995; 105: 30S-6S.
20. Cooper KD, Fox P, Neises G, *et al*. Effects of ultraviolet radiation on human epidermal cell alloantigen presentation: initial depression of Langerhans cell-dependant function is followed by the appearance of T6DR+ cells that enhance epidermal alloantigen presentation. *J Immunol* 1985; 134: 129-37.
21. Kim TY, Kripke ML, Ullrich SE. Immunodepression by factors released from UV-irradiated epidermal cells: selective effects on the generation of contact and delayed hypersensitivity after exposure to UVA or UVB radiation. *J Invest Dermatol* 1990; 94: 26-32.
22. De Fabo EC, Noonan FP. Mechanism of immunosupression by UV irradiation *in vivo*: evidence for the existence of a unique photoreceptors in the skin and its role in photoimmunology. *J Exp Med* 1983; 157: 84-98.
23. Gibbs NK, Norval M, Traynor NJ, Wolf M, Johnson BA, Crosby J. Action spectra for the trans to cis photoisomerization of urocanic acid *in vitro* and in mouse skin. *Photochem Photobiol* 1993; 57: 584-90.
24. Levee GJ, Oberhelman L, Anderson T, Koren H, Cooper KD. UVAII exposure of human skin results in decreased immunization capacity, increased induction of tolerance and a unique pattern of epidermal antigen-presenting cell alteration. *Photochem Photobiol* 1997; 65: 622-9.
25. Streilein JW, Bergstresser PR. Genetic basis of ultraviolet-B effects on contact hypersentivity. *Immunogenetics* 1988; 27: 252-8.
26. Cooper KD, Oberhelman L, Hamilton TA, Baadsgaard O, Terhune M, Levee G, Abderson T, Koren H. UV exposure reduces immunization rates and promotes tolerance to epicutaneous antigens in humans -relationship to dose, CD1a-DR + epidermal macrophage induction, and Langerhans cell depletion. *Proc Natl Acad Sci USA* 1992; 89: 8497-501.
27. Morison WL, Pike RA, Kripke ML. Effect on sunlight and its component wavebands on contact hypersensitivity in mice and guinea-pig. *Photodermatol* 1985; 2: 195-204.
28. Cooper KD. Effects of UV radiation from artificial light sources on the human immune system. *Photochem Photobiol* 1995; 61: 231-5.
29. Yoshikawa T, Rae V, Bruins-Hot W, Vabder Berg JW, Taylor JR, Streilein JW. Susceptibility to effects of UVB radiation on induction of contact hypersensitivity as a risk factor for skin cancer in humans. *J Invest Dermatol* 1990; 95: 530-6.

30. Schwartz. Effects of UVA light on the immune system. A settled issue? *Eur J Dermatol* 1996; 6: 227-8.
31. Van Praag MCG, Out-Luyting C, Claas FHJ, Vermeer BJ, Mommaas AM. Effect of topical sunscreens on the UV-radiation induced suppression of the alloactivating capacity in human skin *in vivo*. *J Invest Dermatol* 1991; 97: 629-33.
32. Wolf P, Kripke ML. Sunscreeens and immunity. *Skin cancer* 1993; 8: 33-40.
33. Wolf P, Donawho CK, Kripke ML. Analysis of the protective effect of different sunscreens on ultraviolet radiation induced local and systemic suppression of contact hypersensitivity and inflammatory responses in mice. *J Invest Dermatol* 1993; 100: 254-9.
34. Whitmore SE, Morison WL. Prevention of UVB induced immunosuppression in humans by a high sun protection factor sunscreen. *Arch Dermatol* 1995; 131: 1128-33.
35. Bestak R, Barnetson RSC, Nearn MR, Halliday GM. Sunscreen protection of contact hypersensitivity. Responses from chronic solar simulated ultraviolet irradiation correlates with the absorption spectrum of the sunscreen. *J Invest Dermatol* 1995; 105: 345-51.
36. Roberts LK, Beasley DG. Commercial sunscreen lotions prevent ultraviolet radiation induced immunosuppression of contact hypersensitivity. *J Invest Dermatol* 1995; 105: 339-44.
37. Hersey P, Mac Donald DM, Burns C, Schibeci S, *et al*. Analysis of the effect of a sunscreen agent on the suppression of Natural Killer Cell activity induced in human subjects by radiation from solarium lamps. *J Invest Dermatol* 1987; 88: 271-6.
38. Fuller CJ, Faulkner H, Bendich A, Parker RS, Roe DA. Effect of β carotene supplementation on photosuppression of delayed type hypersensitivity in normal young men. *Am J Clin Nutr* 1992; 56: 684-90.
39. Uitto J, Brown DB, Gasparro FP, Bernstein EF. Molecular aspects of photoaging. *Eur J Dermatol* 1997; 7: 210-4.
40. Gilchrest BA. Skin aging and photoaging an overview. *J Am Acad Dermatol* 1989; 21: 610-3.
41. Kligman LH, Akin T, Kligman AM. The contributions of UVA and UVB to connective tissue damage in hairless mice. *J Invest Dermatol* 1985; 4: 272-6.
42. Lowe NJ, Meyers DP, Wieder JM, Luftman D, Borget T, Lehman MD, Johnson AW, Scott IR. Low doses of repetitive ultraviolet A induce morphologic changes in human skin. *J Invest Dermatol* 1995; 105: 739-43.
43. Lavker RM, Gerberick GF, Veres DA, Irwin CT, Kaidbey KH. Cumulative effects from repeated exposures to suberythemal doses of UVB and UVA in human skin. *J Am Acad Dermatol* 1995; 32: 53-62.
44. Lavker RM, Veres DA, Irwin CJ, Kaidbey KH. Quantitative assessment of cumulative damage from repetitive exposures to suberythemogenic doses of UVA in human skin. *Photochem Photobiol* 1995; 62: 348-52.
45. Seite S, Moyal D, Richard S, de Rigal J, Leveque JL, Hourseau C, Fourtanier A. Mexoryl® SX: a broad absorption UVA filter protects human skin from the effects of repeated suberythemal doses of UVA J. *Photochem Photobio Biology* 1998; 44: 69-76.
46. Seite S, Piquemal P, Montastier C, Tison-Regnier S, Gueniche A, Christiaens F, Fourtanier A. Effects of repetitive doses of solar simulated UVR in human skin. Protection by a daily use cream. Scientific Poster Contribution. 19th Word Congress of Dermatology –Sydney Australia 1997.
47. Norris PG. Advances in understanding the pathogenesis of photodermatosis. *Curr Op Dermatol* 1993; 1: 185-90.
48. Gonzales E, Gazalez S. Drug photosensitivity, idiopathic photodermatoses and sunscreens. *J Am Acad Dermatol* 1996; 35: 871-85.
49. Gschnait F, Schwarz T, Ladich I. Treatment of polymorphous light eruption. *Arch Dermatol Res* 1983; 275: 379-82.
50. Moyal D, Cesarini JP, Binet O, Hourseau C. Reproduction "in door" de la lucite estivale bénigne. Mise en évidence de l'efficacité d'une crème possédant un fort pouvoir protecteur en UVA. *Nouv Dermatol* 1992; 11: 349-52.
51. Gallen JP, Roth DE, McGrath C, Dromgoole SH. Safety and efficacy of a broad spectrum sunscreen in patients with discoid or subacute cutaneous lupus erythematosus. *Cutis* 1991; 47: 130-6.
52. Farr PM, Diffey BL. Adverses effects of sunscreens in photosensitive patients. *Lancet* 1989; 1: 429-31.

Persistent pigment darkening as a method for the UVA protection assessment of sunscreens

A. Chardon, D. Moyal, C. Hourseau

A. Chardon, D. Moyal, C. Hourseau: L'Oréal, Clichy, France.

Recent studies have shown that even small suberythemogenic amounts of UVA radiation can cause significant chronic photodamage to human skin, at epidermal as well as at dermal level [1, 2]. Thus, there is now a well documented need for UVA protection by sunscreens. The labelling of the sun product efficacy in this waveband calls for an accurate and relevant assessment method in order to supply valuable information to the consumer, in complement to the current SPF number which reflects the efficiency against erythema in UVB and short UVA wavebands.

Existing methods

Many methods, both *in vitro* and *in vivo*, have been proposed to assess the UVA protection efficacy of sunscreens.

In vitro techniques consist in measuring the spectral absorbance of the tested sunscreen in the form of a thin layer, either in solution in a quartz spectrophotometric cell or applied as a film onto a UV transparent substrate like epidermis, skin resin replica or a plastic perforated film with surface structure.

In vivo techniques, either applied to animal or to human skin, consist of applying a series of UVA doses from various solar simulators and observing a quantifiable skin response as an end-point: the number of sunburn cells or the intensity of erythema induced after skin sensitization by anthracene or psoralen derivatives, the unsensitized skin erythema, the Immediate Pigment Darkening (IPD) [3-6], observed immediately post-exposure, and the Persistent Pigment Darkening (PPD), observed 2 to 24 hours post-exposure [3-7]. *In vivo* reflection without UV skin response may also be used.

In vitro techniques are fast and non expensive. Supplying spectral data, they allow mathematical modelling. They do not take into account interactions between products and skin and between wavelengths. Because of the week UVA doses applied onto the product, the photostability of the filtering system is not challenged. Thus, they should not be used for product labelling, since they have not been validated against *in vivo* accepted methodology.

In vivo techniques using erythema developed in photosensitized human skin should only be used for research purposes. They are not relevant for healthy skin users. An *in vivo* method should be based on a actual skin response with an action spectrum covering the whole UVA waveband.

From this point of view, and for ethical reason, the *in vivo* method based on the Immediate Pigment Darkening (IPD) skin response and more specifically on its lasting component, the Persistent Pigment Darkening (PPD), appears strongly recommendable for the UVA protection assessment of sunscreens, because it is non-invasive and relatively easy to perform for routine testing in human.

IPD/PPD skin response

We have investigated the various aspects of the IPD/PPD skin response: action spectra and efficacy spectra, setting up and fading kinetics, dose-response effects at various time lags post-exposure, time-flux reciprocity law.

Action spectra and efficacy spectra

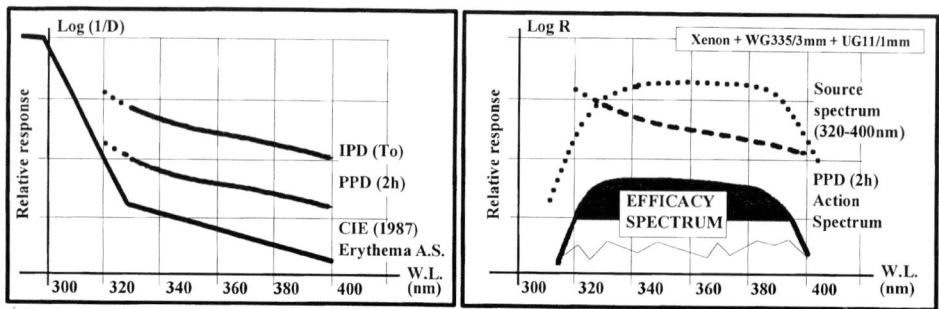

Figure 1. *Action spectra and efficacy spectrum.*

The IPD action spectrum, observed immediately post-exposure, and PPD action spectrum, observed at 2 hours post-exposure, extend over the whole UVA waveband and short visible. UV solar simulator and optical filters must be chosen to ensure that the efficacy spectrum of the end-point is specific for the UVA waveband (320-400 nm).

Kinetics and dose-responses

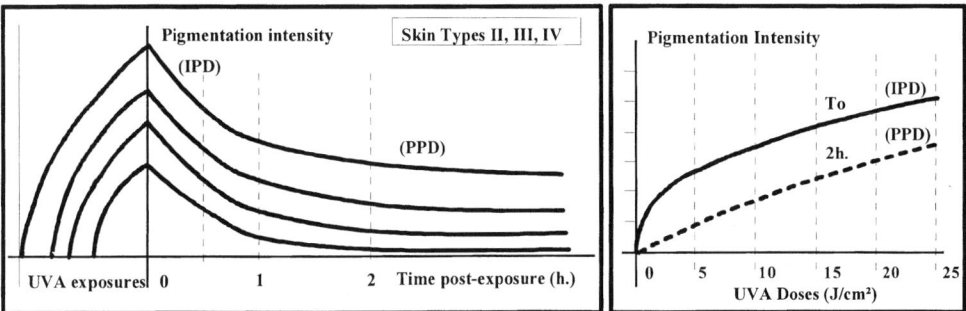

Figure 2. *Kinetics and dose-response of UVA immediate pigmentation (IPD/PPD).*

Immediately during exposure pigmentation developed, reaching its maximal intensity at the end of exposure.
Then a total (low UVA doses) or partial fading (higher UVA doses) occurred rapidly within one hour post-exposure.

For the highest UVA doses, a stable residue was observed which could last several days.
Actually, the "IPD" response would include two main phenomena, the transient phenomenon (IPD) and the persistent one (PPD).
About two hours post-exposure, the dose-response curve of the persistent pigmentation (PPD) is quasi-linear, without significant "threshold".

Reciprocity law (IPD/PPD)

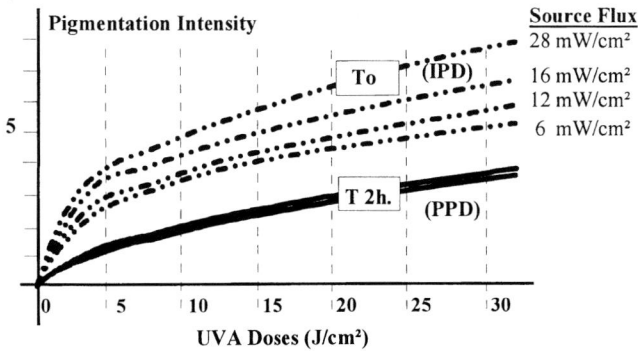

Figure 3. *Reciprocity law for for IPD/PPD skin response.*

The reciprocity law (with equal UV doses (flux x time), equal response intensities are induced, regardless of flux and time) for the unstable IPD response, observed immediately post-exposure appeared to fail, the phenomenon being flux dependent. In contrast, for the stable PPD response, observed at 2 hours post-exposure, the law was fulfilled and the dose-response curves were quasi-linear.

Protocol

The knowledge resulting from the above studies allowed a protocol to be developed for an appropriate UVA-PF test, able to supply reliable, accurate and relevant data.

Table I. *Protocol for a relevant UVA protection factor test method [8]*	
Skin response	Persistent Pigment Darkening (PPD)
Skin type	II, III, IV
UVA dose range	6-30 J/cm² (unprotected skin)
Nb. of doses	6
Progression	25%
UVA source	Xe filtered with WG335/3 mm + UG11/1 mm
Observations	Typically 2 hours – until 24 hours post-exposure
Result	UVA-PF = MPDp/MPDu

MPDp, MPDu: Minimal Pigmenting Doses on protected and unprotected skin.

Note: In applying the "IPD" method for the comparative tests hereafter, the UVA dose range was 1-5 J/cm² and the observation time was within 1 mn post-exposure.

Results

Neutral density physical filters

The methodology was calibrated using neutral density physical filters as standards with respective absorbance values giving nominal UVA-PF values around 4, 8 and 10.
Likely by lack of validity of the reciprocity law (unstable response), the results observed immediately post-exposure with the IPD method, significantly exceeded the nominal values. With the PPD method, the results observed at 2 hours post-exposure were close to the nominal values.

Table II. *UVA-PF (S.D., n) obtained with IPD and PPD methods on calibrated neutral density physical filters*

Nominal value (Spectrophotometric)	IPD (Immediate)	PPD (2 hours)
Std 4	5.3 (1.1, 6)	4.0 (1.3, 8)
Std 8	14.3 (5.4, 6)	6.8 (3.2, 8)
Std 10	21.4 (6.9, 6)	9.0 (3.2, 10)

Sun protective products

Different typical formulations combining UVB and UVA filters were tested with both IPD and PPD techniques.

Table III. *UVA-Protection Factprs (S.D.) of Sun Protective Products Comparison of IPD and PPD methods (n = 10)*

Products Formula (* UVA filters)	End-point (Observation time)	
	IPD (Immediate)	PPD (2 hours)
1% Parsol 1789*	4.8 (1.5)	2.2 (0.5)
3% Parsol 1789*	7.7 (2.4)	4.0 (0.8)
5% Parsol 1789*	13.7 (4.2)	4.6 (1.2)
1% Parsol 1789* 10% Octocrylene	11.1 (3.7)	4.6 (1.0)
3% Parsol 1789* 10% Octocrylene	17.0 (4.1)	8.5 (2.6)
5% Parsol 1789* 10% Octocrylene	39.9 (11.8)	10.6 (2.2)
3.5% Parsol 1789* 3% Mexoryl SX* 3% Mexoryl XL* 10% Octocrylene 5% TiO$_2$	81.3 (16.6)	28.2 (7.0)

The IPD method which uses an unstable response (no compliance with the reciprocity law) lead to an overestimation of the product efficacy.

When UVA doses similar to sun exposure (10-20 J/cm^2 on unprotected skin, equivalent to one hour of sun exposure) are applied with the PPD method, photostability of the sunscreen is taken into account in the UVA protection factor.

Photostabilization of Parsol 1789 by an appropriate UVB filter, Octocrylene [Uvinul N539], clearly improved the UVA protective efficacy of this sunscreen.
Optimal UVA protection was obtained when three complementary effective UVA sunscreens, photostable [Mexoryl® SX and Mexoryl® XL] and photostabilized Parsol 1789, were combined.

Conclusion

Thus, the PPD methodology, drawn up on the basis of extensive colorimetric studies of the complex IPD/PPD phenomenon, based on the residual stable part of this skin response, calibrated with physical neutral density filters and widely used in recent years on numerous actual formulations, could be recognised as the right method for labelling the UVA protection efficacy of sunscreens.

References

1. Lavker R, Gerberick G, Veres D, Irwin C, Kaidbey K. Cumulative effects from repeated exposures to suberythemal doses of UVB and UVA in human skin. *J Am Acad Dermatol* 1995; 32: 53-62.
2. Lowe NJ, Wieder J, Bourget T, Meyers DP, Scott IR, Jonhson AW. Small daily doses of UVA induce major changes in previously unexposed skin within several months. *J Invest Dermatol*, Abstract 230, 1994; vol 103, 435.
3. Roelandts R, Sohrabvand N, Garmyn M. Evaluating the UVA protection of sunscreens. *J Am Acad Dermatol* 1989; 21: 56-62.
4. Cole C, van Fossen R: Measurement of sunscreen UVA protection: an unsensitized human model. *J Am Acad Dermatol* 1992; 26 : 178-84.
5. Poelman MC, Césarini JP, Ruse F, Binet O. A non phototoxic method for testing *in vivo* the UVA photoprotection. XIVth IFSCC Congress (Barcelona). *Preprints* 1986; 2 : 811-3.
6. Kaidbey K, Gange RW. Comparison of methods for assessing photoprotection against UVA *in vivo*. *J Am Acad Dermatol* 1987; 16 : 346-53.
7. Moyal D, Chardon A, Hourseau C. Colorimetric definition of the immediate pigment darkening: its application for the determination of UVA sun-protection-factor. XVI IFSCC Congress (New-York). Poster B22. 10/1990.
8. Japan Cosmetic Industry Association (JCIA): Measurement Standards for UVA protection efficacy. Nov. 21, 1995.

Protection of the Skin against Ultraviolet Radiations
A. Rougier, H. Schaefer, eds. John Libbey Eurotext, Paris © 1998, pp. 137-142

Suncare product photostability: a key parameter for a more realistic *in vitro* efficacy evaluation. Part I: *in vitro* efficacy assessment

B.L. Diffey, R.P. Stokes, S. Forestier, C. Mazilier, A. Richard, A. Rougier

B.L. Diffey, R.P. Stokes: Dryburn Hospital, Durham, United Kingdom.
S. Forestier, C. Mazilier: L'Oréal, Applied Research and Development, Clichy, France.
A. Richard: La Roche-Posay Pharmaceutical Laboratories, 86270 La Roche-Posay, France.
A. Rougier: La Roche-Posay Pharmaceutical Laboratories, Courbevoie, France.

There is little dispute that modern suncare products should provide protection against exposure to both UVB and UVA radiation, and that the product should maintain this broad-spectrum protection throughout the period of exposure to the sun. We have described previously an in vitro methodology for the assessment of suncare product efficacy by transmission spectroscopy [1]. We now describe a modification to the method which takes into account the influence of the exposure of the product to solar ultraviolet (UV) radiation by introducing pre-irradiation prior to the transmission measurements. By this means we can examine the influence of UV exposure on the protection efficacy of the product throughout the ultraviolet spectrum.

Products evaluated

We have applied this new *in vitro* method to evaluate the photostability of nine sunscreen products available in Europe, and which contained the following UV filters.

Method

A micropipette was used to dispense the desired amount of sunscreen onto two quartz plates with roughened surfaces. A light, circular, rubbing motion with a gloved finger was then used to achieve, as uniformly as possible, a 1 mg/cm^2 distribution of sunscreen over the plates.

UV filter	Sunscreen Product								
	A'	B'	C'	D	E	F	G	H	I
MBC	3	3	3	3	-	3	-	-	3
OMC	-	-	-	-	3	-	3	3	3
PBSA	-	-	-	3	-	-	3	-	-
OT	-	-	-	3	-	3	-	-	-
IAMC	-	-	-	3	-	-	-	-	-
HS	-	-	-	-	-	3	-	-	-
OS	-	-	-	-	-	3	-	3	-
BP	-	-	-	-	-	-	-	3	-
BMDM	3	3	3	3	-	3	3	-	3
TDCSA	3	3	3	-	-	-	-	-	-
TiO^2	3	3	3	3	3	3	3	-	3
MICA	-	-	-	-	-	-	3	-	3

Abbreviation

MBC	4-Methylbenzylidene Camphor	OS	Octyl Salicylate
OMC	Octyl Methoxycinnamate	BP	Benzophenone-3
PBSA	Phenylbenzimidazole Sulfonic Acid	BMDM	Butyl Methoxydibenzoylmethane
OT	Octyl Triazone		
IAMC	Isoamyl p-Methoxycinnamate	TDCSA	Terephthalylidene Dicamphor Sulfonic Acid
HS	Homosalate		
TiO$_2$	Titanium Dioxide	MICA	Mica

Initially, both plates were placed inside a dark oven set at 30 ± 2° C for 15 minutes to allow the sunscreen to dry. Both plates were removed from the oven and one of them, the *test plate*, fixed to a specially-designed holder which allowed spectral transmission measurements to be carried out, as well as irradiation with solar simulating radiation. *In vitro* assessment of sunscreen protection was measured on both the test and control plates and the SPF calculated [1].

The *control plate* was returned to the oven, whilst the test plate was positioned 12 cm in front of the exit port of a solar simulator which comprised a 900 W Xe arc lamp filtered by UG5 (1 mm) and WG320 (1 mm) glass filters, giving an unweighted UV irradiance of 5.2 ± 0.3 mW/cm^2.

At times of 75, 135 and 195 minutes after product application, both plates were removed from their respective positions and SPF measurements repeated. Thus the test plate received doses of 18, 36 and 54 J/cm^2. The whole process was repeated three times for each product.

Results

Table I gives the mean SPFs of each sunscreen product as a function of time after the initial 15 minutes drying time, for the irradiated and control samples. In order to compare whether there was a difference between the two samples with time, a normalized area under the curve (NAUC) was calculated for each serial measurement on a given sample and compared using an unpaired t-test [2].

We can see that products A, C, F and H appear photostable, products B and E exhibit minor photodegradation, whilst products D, G and I show marked reduction in SPF with irradiation. *Figure 1* shows the change in SPF with UV dose for each of the nine products.

To investigate the change in UVA absorption of the products, we calculated the ratio of the mean UVA absorbance to the mean UVB absorbance, which is defined as:

$$\Re = \frac{\int_{320}^{400} A(\lambda)d\lambda / \int_{320}^{400} d\lambda}{\int_{290}^{320} A(\lambda)d\lambda / \int_{290}^{320} d\lambda}$$

Table I. Mean SPFs on each sample						
Product		Duration of exposure (thermal or UV), hours				P-value or difference in photostability
		0	1	2	3	
A	Control	58	57	57	55	0.47
	Test	56	53	55	50	
B	Control	25	26	25	25	0.009
	Test	29	28	27	26	
C	Control	33	31	31	30	0.32
	Test	30	30	30	29	
D	Control	65	62	59	55	< 0.0001
	Test	65	32	30	29	
E	Control	18	18	18	17	0.03
	Test	18	16	15	13	
F	Control	41	41	43	42	0.07
	Test	43	41	41	39	
G	Control	24	24	22	22	< 0.0001
	Test	22	12	10	9	
H	Control	18	18	18	18	0.21
	Test	17	17	17	16	
I	Control	38	37	36	35	< 0.0001
	Test	33	13	11	9	

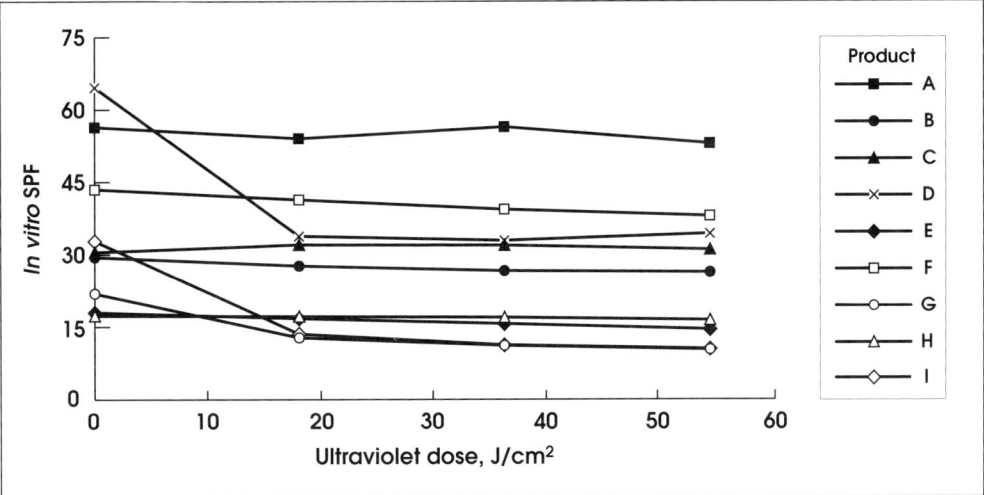

Figure 1. In vitro *SPF on each product corrected for thermal effects.*

where $A(\lambda)$ is the effective absorbance and related to the sunscreen transmittance $T(\lambda)$ by $A(\lambda) = -\log[T(\lambda)]$. The absorbance ratio will range from 0 for products exhibiting no protection against UVA radiation to 1 for products exhibiting equal absorption at all wavelengths through the UV spectrum. The mean NAUC for the irradiated and control samples were again compared using an unpaired t-test *(Table II)*. Products E and H appear photostable, products A, B, C, and F exhibit a mild reduction in UVA protection, and products D, G and I show marked reduction in UVA stability with irradiation.

Table II. *Mean UVA: UVB absorbance ratios on each sample*

Product		Duration of exposure (thermal or UV), hours				P-value or difference in photostability
		0	1	2	3	
A	Control	0.76	0.76	0.76	0.75	0.001
	Test	0.77	0.74	0.73	0.71	
B	Control	0.68	0.68	0.68	0.68	0.0025
	Test	0.68	0.66	0.65	0.64	
C	Control	0.72	0.71	0.71	0.71	0.0084
	Test	0.71	0.70	0.68	0.67	
D	Control	0.45	0.44	0.43	0.42	0.0001
	Test	0.44	0.30	0.30	0.29	
E	Control	0.40	0.40	0.41	0.41	0.0038
	Test	0.37	0.40	0.42	0.42	
F	Control	0.57	0.57	0.57	0.57	0.0037
	Test	0.56	0.54	0.53	0.52	
G	Control	0.54	0.54	0.53	0.52	0.0004
	Test	0.53	0.40	0.39	0.41	
H	Control	0.44	0.45	0.45	0.45	0.78
	Test	0.45	0.46	0.46	0.46	
I	Control	0.63	0.63	0.63	0.62	< 0.0001
	Test	0.61	0.36	0.33	0.33	

Discussion

We found that the SPFs and UVA:UVB absorbance ratios remained stable when the active ingredients contained photostable UV filtering systems (eg Butyl Methoxydibenzoylmethane/4-Methylbenzylidene Camphor/Terephthalylidene Dicamphor Sulfonic Acid). In contrast, with photo-unstable ingredients, the protection indices dropped significantly following UV exposure. For example, UV filtering systems containing Butyl Methoxydibenzoylmethane/Octyl Methoxycinnamate suffered protection efficacy losses up to 50-60% of their initial value. The addition of photo-stabilizing UV filtering systems did not prevent these reductions in protection efficacy.

Our observations reveal that the most important variations of the photoprotective efficacy of unstable products occur during the first 60 minutes of the UV exposure. Thus, *Figure 2* shows the changes in UV transmission of the nine products, before and after such an exposure, for the global UV radiation, the short wavelength ($\lambda < 350$ nm) and the long wavelength ($\lambda > 350$ nm) UVA radiations. Each graph bar describes the percentage of UV light transmitted through the sunscreen product film [3]: this unabsorbed part of the UV light is in fact the

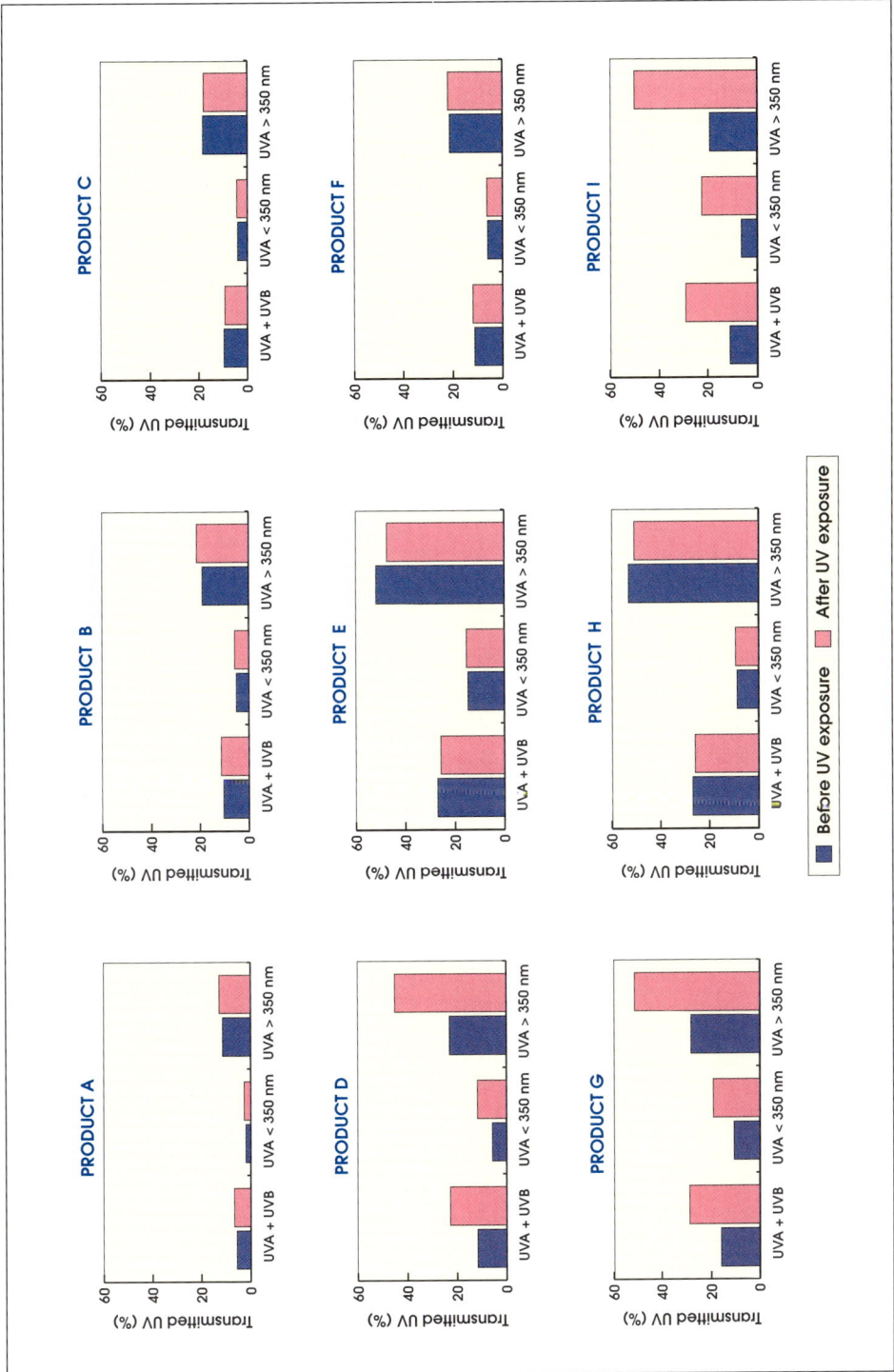

Figure 2. Transmitted UV percentages before and after a 60 min UV exposure.

most important, as only unfiltered UV radiation will be responsible of deleterious effects. In such graphs, when an increase of the transmitted UV percentage is observed, it translates the photo-unstability of the sunscreen product. An ideal sunscreen would be a product which has both qualities of highly filtering system and a good photostability: the results in *Figure 2* clearly show that only the products A, B, C and F fulfill these two requirements.

Conclusion

This study has demonstrated the importance of taking into account the photostability of suncare products when evaluating their protection efficacy by an *in vitro* technique. With sample pre-irradiation, it is possible to evaluate the efficacy of suncare products in more realistic experimental conditions akin to their use *in vivo*.

* Product A: ANTHELIOS L; Product B: ANTHELIOS S; Product C: ANTHE-LIOS 20B.

References

1. Diffey BL, Robson J. A new substrate to measure sunscreen protection factors throughout the ultraviolet spectrum. J Soc Cosmet Chem 1989; 40: 127-33.
2. Matthews JNS, Altman DG, Campbell MJ, Royston P. Analysis of serial measurements in medical research. BMJ 1990; 300: 230-5.
3. Marginean G, Fructus AE, Marty JP, Arnaud-Battandier J. New ex-vivo method for evaluating the photoprotective efficacy of sunscreens. Intern J Cosmet Sci 1995; 17: 233-44.

Suncare product photostability: a key parameter for a more realistic *in vitro* efficacy evaluation. Part II: chromatographic analysis

S. Forestier, C. Mazilier, A. Richard, A. Rougier

S. Forestier, C. Mazilier: L'Oréal, Applied Research and Development, Clichy, France.
A. Richard: La Roche-Posay Pharmaceutical Laboratories, 86270 La Roche-Posay, France.
A. Rougier: La Roche-Posay Pharmaceutical Laboratories, Courbevoie, France.

During recent years, there has been an increased awareness of the potentially damaging effects of UVA radiation to human skin. This has lead to the development of suncare products providing good protection against UVA radiation, associated to high photoprotective level against UVB radiation. As the consumer is becoming used to being exposed for longer periods in the sun, it has become mandatory that the UV filters ensuring the product efficacy remain chemically unaltered by sun radiation, throughout the sunlight exposure. Thus, suncare product photostability has arisen as a major requirement for broad spectrum protection.

Various in vitro methodologies have been proposed for the evaluation of the photochemical stability of organic UV filters in suncare products, for example using photometric [1] or spectroradiometric [2] transmission measurements. But such methods can be affected by optical artefacts, such as photoproducts which absorb in the UV range. Therefore, chromatographic analysis of residual amounts of sunfilters after UV exposure [3] is mandatory for appreciating the product photostability, as the loss of some organic filters, due to their photodegradation, will reduce the product efficacy. Such an analysis can assess the particular interest of some UV filters associations, which have been proved to be unsensitive to sunlight exposure.

We describe below an in vitro methodology for the assessment of suncare product photostability, using post exposure chromatographic analysis of UV filters, in addition to optical transmission measurements.

Products evaluated

This methodology was tested by assessing the photostability of nine suncare products of the european market, which protection efficacy alterations under UV exposure have been otherwise tested [2].

Method

Sunscreen product was applied using a spatula on two polymethylmethacrylate plates with roughened surface. The product was then spread with the spatula on a well defined 8 cm^2 area in the middle of the plate, as uniformly as possible, in order to obtain a 2 mg/cm^2 distribution of the sunscreen to be tested. This amount of applied product has been chosen to allow the chromatographic analysis after UV exposure to be performed with a good level of accuracy, even when UV filter photodegradation occurs.

UV filter	Sunscreen Product								
	A'	B'	C'	D	E	F	G	H	I
MBC	✓	✓	✓	✓	-	✓	-	-	✓
OMC	-	-	-	-	✓	-	✓	✓	✓
PBSA	-	-	-	✓	-	-	✓	-	-
OT	-	-	-	✓	-	✓	-	-	-
IAMC	-	-	-	✓	-	-	-	-	-
HS	-	-	-	-	-	✓	-	-	-
OS	-	-	-	-	-	✓	-	✓	-
BP	-	-	-	-	-	-	-	✓	-
BMDM	✓	✓	✓	✓	-	✓	✓	-	✓
TDCSA	✓	✓	✓	-	-	-	-	-	-
TiO$_2$	3	✓	✓	✓	✓	✓	✓	-	✓
MICA	-	-	-	-	-	-	✓	-	✓

Abbreviation

MBC	4-Methylbenzylidene Camphor
OMC	Octyl Methoxycinnamate
PBSA	Phenylbenzimidazole Sulfonic Acid
OT	Octyl Triazone
IAMC	Isoamyl p-Methoxycinnamate
HS	Homosalate
OS	Octyl Salicylate
BP	Benzophenone-3
BMDM	Butyl Methoxydibenzoylmethane
TDCSA	Terephthalylidene Dicamphor Sulfonic Acid
TiO2	Titanium Dioxide
MICA	Mica

Table I. *Residual UV filters after UV exposure*

Product	Percentage of recovery of UV filters after UV exposure (12 J/cm^2)									
	MBC	OMC	PBSA	OT	IAMC	HS	OS	BP	BMDM	TDCSA
A	91 ± 1	-	-	-	-	-	-	-	85 ± 1	99 ± 1
B	97 ± 2	-	-	-	-	-	-	-	85 ± 4	98 ± 2
C	94 ± 1	-	-	-	-	-	-	-	93 ± 2	98 ± 3
D	90 ± 1	-	100 ± 2	100 ± 2	56 ± 1	-	-	-	2 ± 1	-
E	-	80 ± 4	-	-	-	-	-	-	-	-
F	98 ± 1	-	-	100 ± 2	-	87 ± 3	83 ± 3	-	90 ± 2	-
G	-	49 ± 4	100 ± 2	-	-	-	-	-	1 ± 1	-
H	-	87 ± 3	-	-	-	-	77 ± 5	94 ± 4	-	-
I	98 ± 3	54 ± 2	-	-	-	-	-	-	9 ± 2	-

Initially, both plates *(control plate and test plate)* were placed inside a dark and ventilated oven set at 40 ± 2° C during 15 minutes to allow the sunscreen films to dry. The control plate was maintained in the oven for the whole duration of the test plate UV exposure.

The test plate was positioned in an HERAEUS Suntest at 23 cm in front of the lamp. Thus, the product on this plate was submitted to a continuous UV irradiation with an unweighted irradiance of 3.5 ± 0.5 mW/cm^2, at a temperature of 40 ± 2° C.

After one hour of UV exposure (equivalent to a 12 J/cm^2 UV dose), the test plate was removed from the Suntest, and the control plate from the oven. Residual filters were extracted from each sunscreen film with 50 ml of methanol. The resulting solutions were analyzed by isocratic HPLC, using a reverse phase C18 column (Merck LiChroSpher 250 x 4 mm 5 µm) and a diode-array detector (Waters 996), with adequate eluent composition for each UV filter to be analyzed.

The whole process was repeated three times on each sunscreen product, and the results were expressed as the mean values of the three samples.

Results

The following table gives the mean percentages of each UV filter in the suncare products recovered one hour after the initial 15 minutes drying time, for the irradiated samples. The analysis of the control samples showed no variation of sunfilter amounts in the samples.

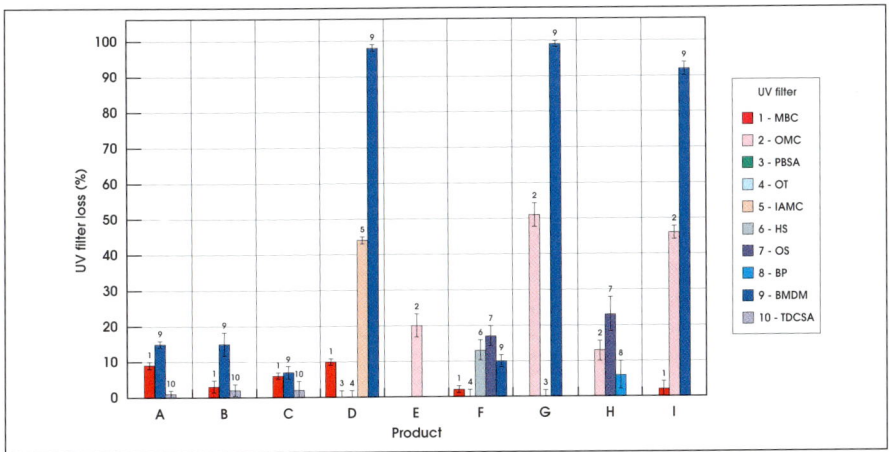

Figure 1. *Loss in UV filters after UV exposure.*

Discussion

Our experiments clearly show losses of some UV filters, due to their photo-unstability. Butyl Methoxydibenzoylmethane is known as a very photo-unstable filter [3]. Similarly Cinnamate and Salicylate derivatives are described as poorly photostable filters. Moreover, in opposition to some previous assertions [4], it is obvious that the combination of Cinnamic Acid esters with Butyl Methoxydibenzoylmethane does not limit the photodegradation of this UVA filter. This explains the important loss observed for Butyl Methoxydibenzoylmethane in products D, G and I. Such a loss will induce dramatic reduction in product efficacy [2].

In contrast, the results confirm that Phenylbenzimidazole Sulfonic Acid, Octyl Triazone, Benzophenone-3 and Terephthalylidene Dicamphor Sulfonic Acid are not affected by UV radiation. This contributes to maintain the photoprotective efficacy of the suncare product throughout the exposure.
It is also shown that the photodegradation of Butyl Methoxydibenzoylmethane can be strongly reduced by involving this filter in photostabilized formulations. Such a decrease in its sensitivity to UV light can be obtained either by stabilizing filters (eg 4-Methylbenzylidene Camphor) and/or by adequate formulating systems. This is specifically illustrated by products A, B and C which have filtering systems that associate Butyl Methoxydibenzoylmethane with 4-Methylbenzylidene Camphor and Terephthalylidene Dicamphor Sulfonic Acid: these two filters contribute to decrease Butyl Methoxydibenzoylmethane photo-unstability and to obtain high levels of photoprotection. With regard to its filtering system composition, product F seems to associate photostabilizing effects, both from the UV filters combination and from appropriate formulation ingredients. Due to low UV filter losses, these products keep their photoprotective efficacy throughout UV exposure [2].

Recently some authors [5] suggested that sunscreen product photostability will no longer be an issue, as far as meaningful protocols for *in vitro* determination of photoprotection are going to be established, which take photostability into account. But it is known that the UV-induced alterations of organic UV filters can go well beyond simple molecular reorganization processes: for the most commonly used UVA filter, Butyl Methoxydibenzoylmethane, they may lead to photoproducts with very poor protective efficacy [6]. Thus, we think that guaranteing the stability of the filtering system throughout UV exposure is a minimal requirement for any suncare product, in order to provide optimal protective efficacy without increasing its cost.

Conclusion

The present study demonstrates the interest of determining the rate of photodegradation of UV filters, following a UV exposure, in order to take into account the sunscreen product photostability when evaluating its protection efficacy by an *in vitro* technique. The chromatographic data are in good agreement with the optical measurements reported elsewhere [2]. In addition, they can explain the reduction of protective efficacy which affect photo-unstable products during UV exposure. By combining these two techniques, suncare product manufacturers can select the most reliable sunfilters to obtain highly protective and photostable products.

* Product A: ANTHELIOS L; Product B: ANTHELIOS S; Product C: ANTHE-LIOS 20B.

> **Acknowledgements**
>
> The authors wish to thank Mrs Lagoutte and Mr Bover who performed the experiments.

References

1. Forestier S, Lang G, Mazilier C. La photostabilité des filtres solaires au service de la durabilité de la protection. IFSCC In-Between Meeting 1995 Montreux.
2. Diffey BL, Stockes RP, Forestier S, Mazilier C, Rougier A. Suncare product photostability: A key parameter for a more realistic *in vitro* efficacy evaluation – Part I : *In vitro* efficacy assessment. 19th World Congress of Dermatology 1997 Sydney.
3. Deflandre A, Lang G. Photostability of sunscreens: Benzylidene camphor and dibenzoylmethane derivatives. *Intern J Cosmet Sci* 1988; 10: 53-62.
4. Shaath NA. Photochemistry and photostability of sunscreen components, mixtures and products. FDA Workshop Photochemistry and Photobiology of Sunscreens 1996 Rockville Maryland.
5. Gonzenbach HU, Pittet GH. Photostability, a must? International Conference "Broadspectrum Sun Protection: The Issues and Status" 1997 London.
6. Rudolph T, Schwack W. Photochemistry of dibenzoylmethane UVA filters in commercial sunscreen products. International Meeting "Photostability of Drugs" 1995 Oslo.

Protection of the Skin against Ultraviolet Radiations
A. Rougier, H. Schaefer, eds. John Libbey Eurotext, Paris © 1998, pp. 149-157

Which kind of protection a broad absorption UVA sunscreen provide?

A. Fourtanier, C. Cohen, A. Guéniche, R. Ley, D. Moyal, S. Seité

A. Fourtanier, C. Cohen, A. Guéniche, S. Seité: Life Sciences, L'Oréal Advanced Research Laboratories, Clichy, France.
D. Moyal: L'Oréal Applied Research and Development, Clichy, France.
R. Ley: The Lovelace Institutes, Albuquerque, USA.

Objective

To test the protection provided or added by a UVA filter offering a broad UV absorption spectrum, such as Mexoryl®SX, against UV induced damage in animal and human skin.

Chemical and physical characteristics of Mexoryl®SX

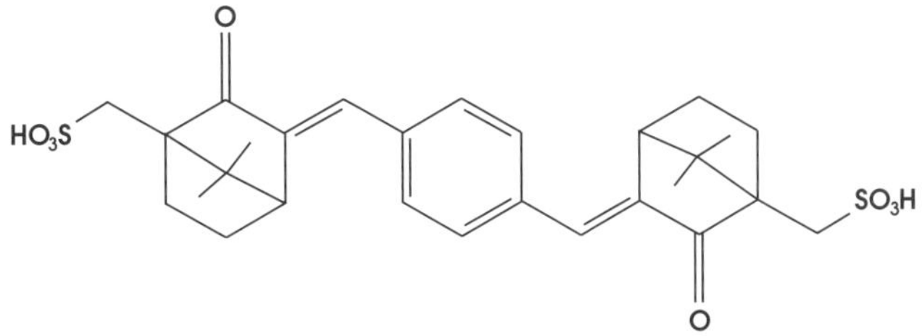

Terephthalylidene Dicamphor Sulfonic Acid

$C_{28}H_{34}O_8S_2$
Molecular weight : 562.3

Σ max = 45.000 M^{-1} cm^{-1}
U.V. (water) : λ max = 345 nm

Figure 1. *Chemical characteristics of Mexoryl®SX.*

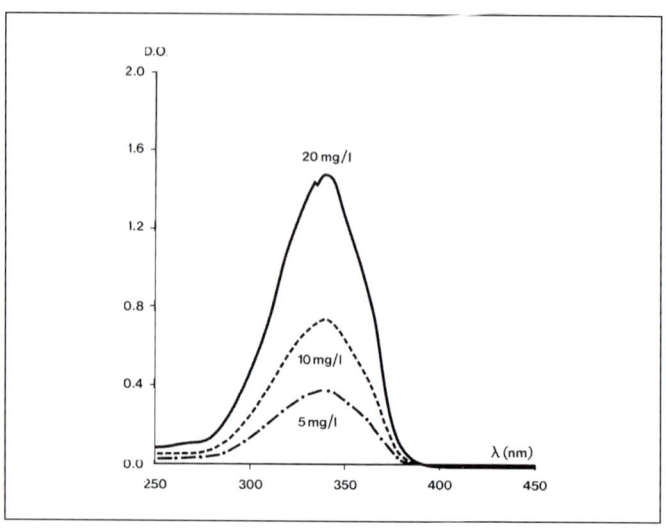

Figure 2. *Physical characteristics of Mexoryl®SX.*

Mexoryl®SX containing formulas protect against drug induced phototoxicity

Two sunscreen formulas were tested for their capacity to protect a reconstructed epidermis (Episkin) from the phototoxic reaction induced by UVA exposure (70 j/cm^2) + chlorpromazine (50 nmol/epidermal equivalent).

Formula A: (SPF = 25 – PPD (UVA) = 5) containing Mexoryl®SX and titanium dioxide.
Formula B: (SPF = 60 – PPD (UVA) = 12) containing Mexoryl®SX – PARSOL®1789 – EUSOLEX®6300 and titanium dioxide.

UVA source: Xenon arc fitted with 2 Schott filters (UG11/1 mm + WG335/3 mm).

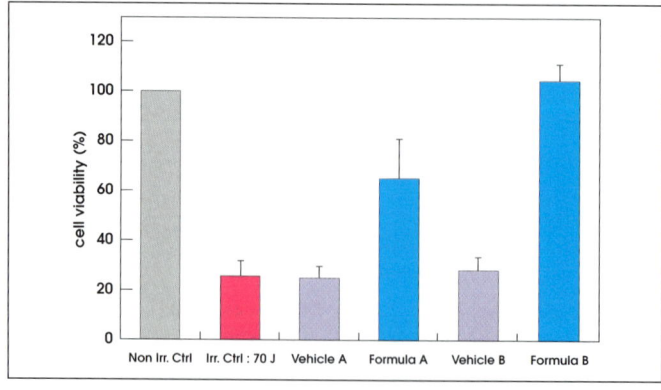

Figure 3. *Test of two sunscreens formulas.*

Mexoryl®SX containing formulas protect against lipoperoxidation induced by UVA

Lipid peroxides were induced in Episkin using a non cytotoxic UVA exposure dose (50 J/cm^2) delivered by the same UVA source as the one used in the phototoxicity test. Generated peroxides were measured using a colorimetric test (LPO – CC – Kamiya Biomedical Company). The same sunscreen formulas A and B were evaluated and compared to two other formulas without Mexoryl®SX.

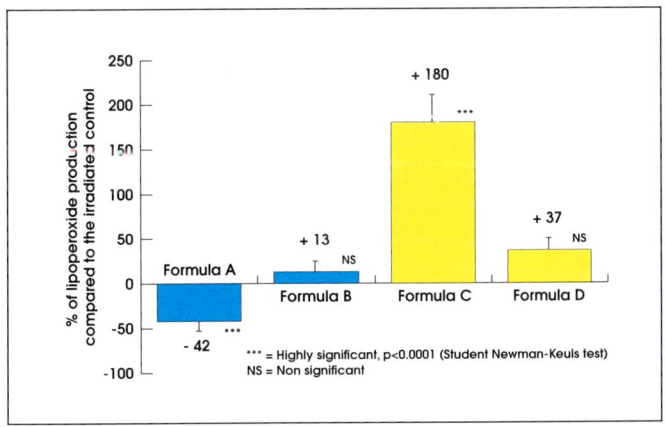

Topical application of 5% Mexoryl®SX provides greater protection (p < 0.05) against solar simulated UVR (SSUV, 290-400 nm) induced pyrimidine dimers than 5% 2-ethylhexyl p-methoxycinnamate (2 EHMC), a UVB absorber

Pyrimidine dimers were measured in epidermal DNA of SKH-HR1 mice following exposure to solar simulated UVR (Xenon arc fitted with Schott filters: UG11/1 mm + WG320/1 mm). The rates of induction of endonuclease sensitive sites (ESS) per 10^8 daltons of basal DNA in untreated (●), vehicle treated (■) 5% 2-EHMC treated (▼) and 5% Mexoryl®SX treated (▲) mice are present on the above graph.

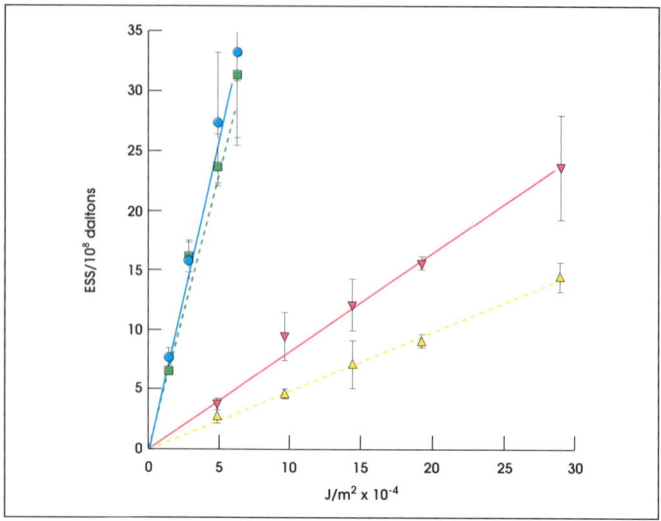

5% Mexoryl®SX is significantly more effective than 5% of 2-ethylhexyl p-methoxycinnamate (2 EHMC), a UVB absorber, in the prevention of systemic suppression of contact hypersensitivity (CHS) to dinitrofluorobenzene (DNCB), induced by solar simulated UVR exposure

Acute exposure to UVR causes immunosuppression of CHS to DNFB a contact sensitizing agent, first applied to a distant unirradiated site (induction) and reapplied on an unirradiated ear (challenge). The immune reaction is evaluated by measurement of ear swelling using a micrometer. Both preparations provided a Sun Protection Factor (SPF) against erythema of about 4.

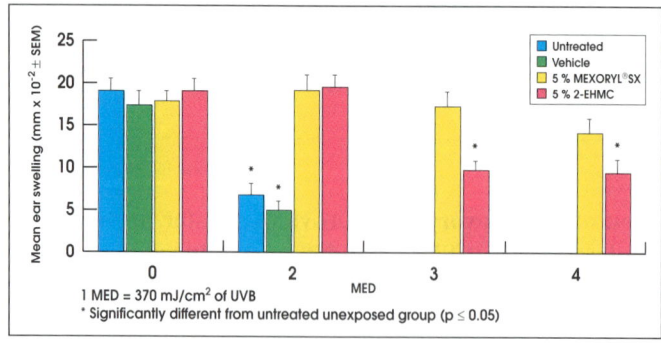

This superiority of Mexoryl®SX containing product can be explained by a better protection of Langerhans cells number and a lower increasedof sera IL-10 production

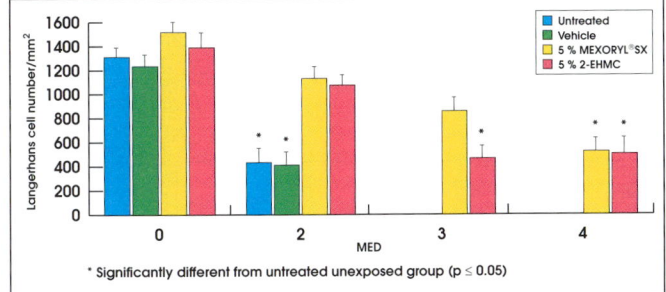

Figure 4. Effect of sunscreens on UVR Langerhans cell depression. Evaluation was done on epidermal sheets using immunoperoxydase staining. N = 10; data are means ± SEM.

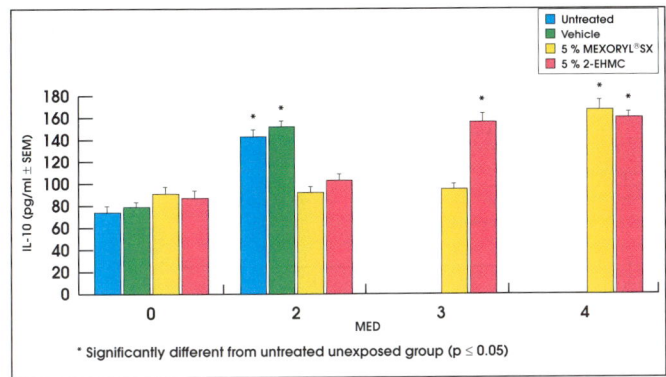

Figure 5. Effect of sunscreens on UVR-induced IL-10 (sera). Evaluation of IL-10 serum level using an ELISA test. N = 10; data are means ± SEM.

Mexoryl®SX protects against solar simulated UVR induced photocarcinogenesis in SKH:HR1 mice. It delays tumor appearance longer than does 2 EHMC (a UVB absorber)

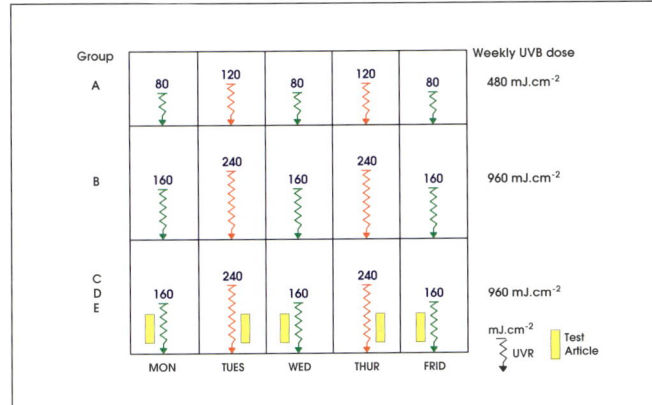

Figure 6. Study design and treatment schedule:
group A = low UVR dose,
group B = high UVR dose,
group C = high UVR dose + 5% Mexoryl®SX,
group D = high UV dose + 10% Mexoryl®SX,
group E = high UVR dose + 5% 2-EHMC.
Each of the five experimental groups contained 28 mice. The cumulative UVR dose delivered on Monday + Wednesday + Friday was equal to the cumulative dose delivered on Tuesday + Thursday. The UVR exposures and the topical applications were performed 5 days per week, Monday through Friday, for 40 weeks followed by a 10 weeks follow-up period with no treatment and no exposure. The UV source was a Xenon solar simulator.

To determine, for regulatory purposes, the potential of Mexoryl®SX to modifiy the UV radiation induced murine skin tumor development and growth, we used a standardized protocol recommended by the Food and Drug Administration.

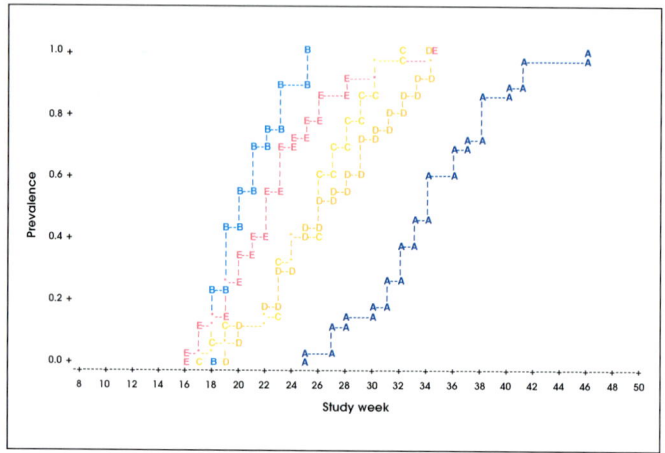

Figure 7. *Kaplan-Meier mortality-free prevalence plots (tumors ≥ 1 mm):*
group A = low UVR dose,
group B = high UVR dose,
group C = high UVR dose + 5% Mexoryl®SX,
group D = high UVR dose + 10% Mexoryl®SX,
group E = high UVR dose + 5% 2-EHMC.

Mexoryl®SX containing formulations are very efficient in Polymorphous Light Eruption prevention (PMLE)

Human female prone to PLE were exposed for 7 days to the Tunisia sun (Djerba). Half body comparisons were performed with 3 different sunscreens (T_1 versus T_2 and T_2 versus T_3). After each exposure (end of the day) a dermatologist scored the clinical signs of PMLE (papules, reticulated erythema or vesicles).

Formulas	SUNSCREEN COMPOSITION						PROTECTION FACTORS	
	UVB FILTERS			UVA FILTERS		MICRO PIGMENTS		
	EUSOLEX® 6300	UVINUL® N539	PARSOL® MCX	PARSOL® 1789	MEXORYL® SX	TiO2	SPF	UVA PF
T_1	●	●	●				15	1
T_2		●		●	●	●	40	6
T_3		●		●	●	●	> 40	>10

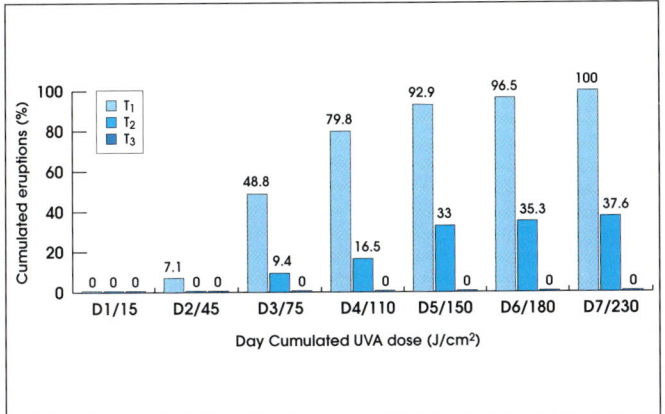

Figure 8. With T_2, the onset of PMLE was either prevented or delayed with a lower intensity in 36 patients out of 43 (84%). With T_3 no incidence of PMLE was observed.

A sunscreen containing 5% Mexoryl®SX is able to prevent or reduce alterations by repeated doses of UVA in mouse and human skin

Mouse study

Two months old SKH-HR1 were exposed for 1 year to suberythemal dose (35 J/cm^2) of UVA with or without the sunscreen. On skin biopsies sampled at the end of the study we observed changes in elastic network using scanning electron microscopy on autoclaved dermis.

Age-associated changes in elastin have been noted at the dermal-epidermal junction (DEJ = yellow dashed line on photographs); the caracteristic candelabra-like organization of fine fibers (blue lines on photographs) could no longer be detected, whereas elastic fibers cylindrical in shape and vertically arranged appeared more compact because of a decrease in spaces

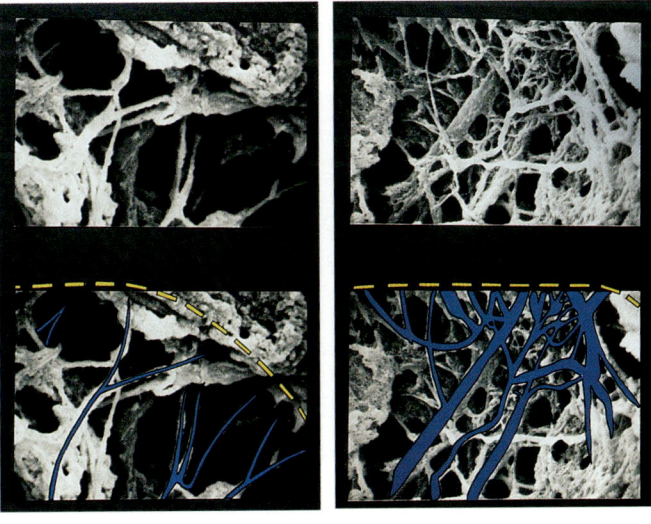

2 months control   14 months control

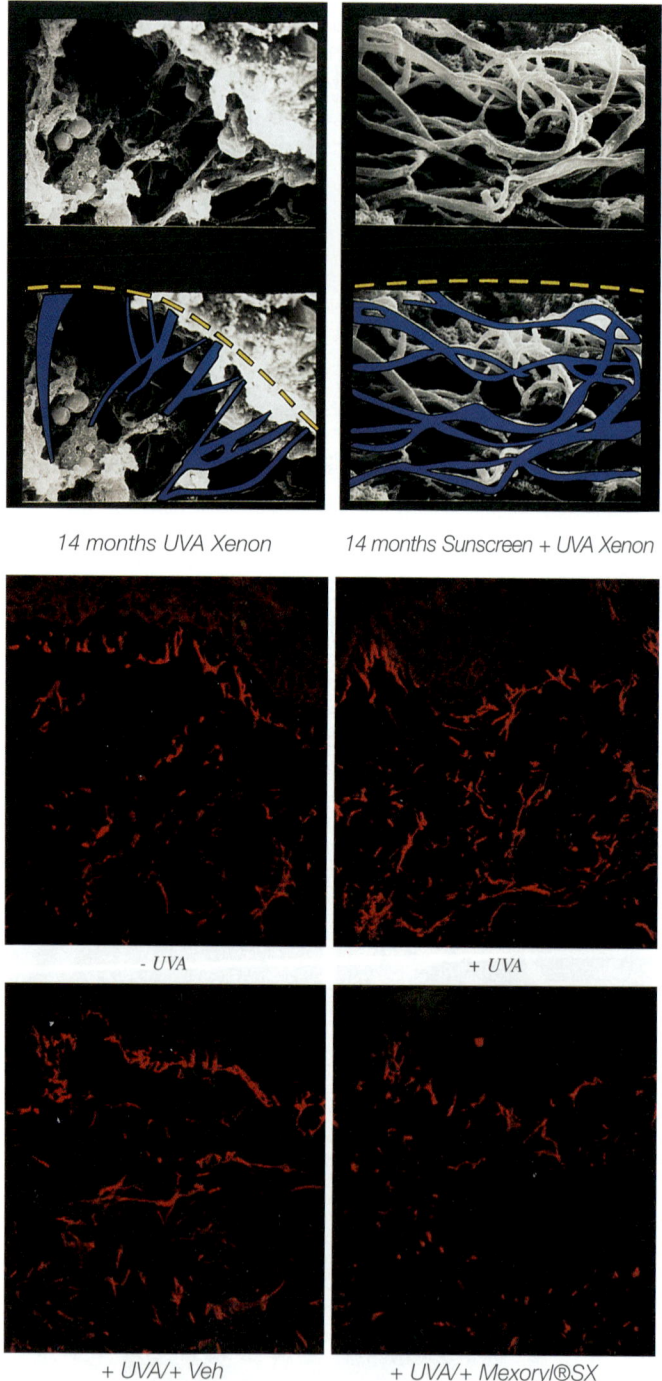

14 months UVA Xenon   *14 months Sunscreen + UVA Xenon*

- UVA   *+ UVA*

+ UVA/+ Veh   *+ UVA/+ Mexoryl®SX*

An increased deposition of lysozyme was seen on + UVA and + UVA + vehicle treated sites. Mexoryl®SX prevents this alteration.

between the fibers. In irradiated groups the orientation of these thicker fibers became parallel to the DEJ. When animals were irradiated and treated with sunscreen, the fibers became compact and thick but they did not lose the vertical arrangement observed in unirradiated animals.

Human study

Three areas of the back of female volunteers were exposed thrice weekly with increasing doses of UVA for 13 weeks. One received the sunscreen prior to exposure (+ UVA/+ Mexoryl®SX), another the vehicle (+ UVA/+ Veh) while the third one was kept untreated (+ UVA). At the end of the study, biopsies were sampled on the 3 exposed sites and on an unexposed control site (– UVA).

Conclusion

These findings suggest that sunscreen products should provide protection throughout the entire UVB + UVA spectrum. Mexoryl®SX which absorbs from 290 up to 400 nm significantly contributes to the improvement of sunscreen efficacy.

Effects of repetitive doses of solar simulated UVR in human skin. Protection by a daily use cream

S. Seité, P. Piquemal, C. Montastier, S. Tison-Regnier, A. Guéniche,
F. Christiaens, A. Fourtanier

S. Seité, S. Tison-Regnier, A. Guéniche, F. Christiaens, A. Fourtanier: Life Sciences, L'Oréal Advanced Research Laboratories, Clichy, France.
P. Piquemal, C. Montastier: L'Oréal, Applied Research and Development, Chevilly-Larue, France.

During normal daily activities an appropriate protection against solar exposure should prevent clinical and cellular changes leading to photoaging, photoimmunosuppression and eventually photocarcinogenesis [1]. This study was designed to evaluate on humans the efficacy of a cream for daily use containing a photostable combination of sunscreens: octocrylene, PARSOL, 1789 and Mexoryl® SX (SPF 8) providing a continuous absorption through the entire UV spectrum.

Materials and methods

Volunteers

12 healthy caucasian males and females – 20 to 35 years old – skin type II and IIIA.

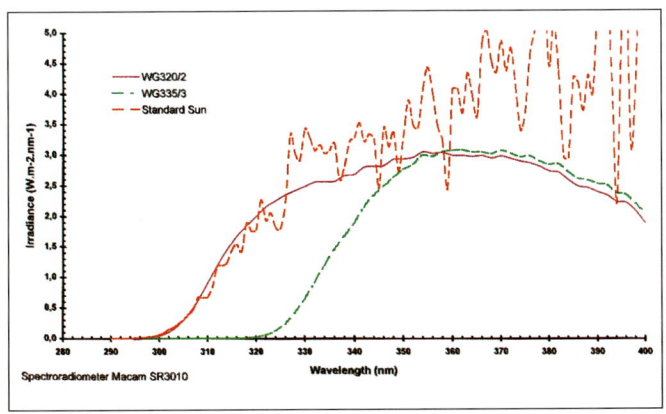

UVR source

An Oriel® 1000 watt xenon arc solar simulator equipped with a Schott® WG320/2 mm filter (300-400 nm) or with a WG335/3 mm (320-400 nm).

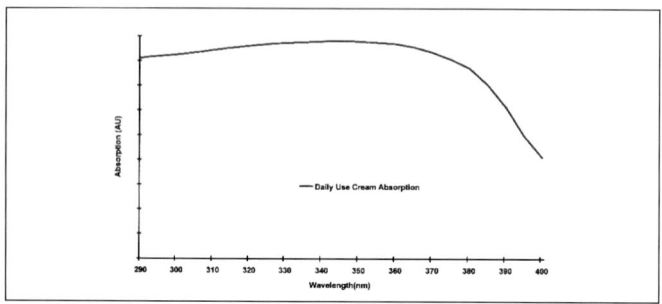

Test products

Vehicle; O/W emulsion based on Arlacel 165. -Daily use cream (= SS): same emulsion containing 1.5% PARSOL, 1789, 1.5% MEXORYL® SX (A.M.) and 4% octocrylene. The Sun Protection Factor (SPF) and the UVA Protection Factor (Persistent Pigmentation Darkening – PPD) were determined on the same volunteers and were 8.39 ± 1.22 (SPF) and 7.4 ± 2.4 (PPD), respectively.

	Med and daily doses of UVB and UVA applied			
		Daily exposure (J/cm²)		
	Med (min)	UVB	UVA	UVA/UVB
Phototypes II + IIIA (n = 12)	9.33 ± 0.37	0.86 ± 0.06	11.05 ± 0.55	13 ± 0.3

Data are mean ± SEM.

Treatments and exposure regimens

4 areas were delineated with a template on the buttock of the volunteers: one area received no exposure and no product was applied (Control). The three others were irradiated 5 days per week for 6 weeks, with one Minimal Erythemal Dose (MED) of Solar Simulated Radiation (SSR) supplemented with UVA to slightly augment the UVA/UVB ratio from 12 to 13 (the standard sun ratio being higher than 16). One area was irradiated untreated (+SSR); one was treated 30 mn before exposure with 2 mg/cm² of vehicle (+SSR/+Veh) and one with 2 mg/cm² of the daily use cream (+SSR/+SS). The total dose delivered was 30 MED.

Antisera	Supplier	Working Dilution
Epidermis		
Ki-67	Daloo	1/200
Dermis		
Factor XIII-A	Nardic	1/100
Vimentin	Manosan	1/100
Tenascin	Chemicon	1/10
Pro-collagen I	Chemicon	1/100
Elastin	IPL	1/50
Lysozyme	Zymed	Undiluted
a-1 antitrypsin	Immunon	Undiluted

Assessments

Clinical and biophysical assessments of erythema, pigmentation and hydration were performed each week. Skin microtopography was evaluated at day 0 and day 8. Biopsy specimens were obtained after the last exposure (day 43 – week 7). Histological evaluations of epidermal (stratum corneum and stratum granulosum thickness, melanization) and dermal (collagen and elastin) parameters were performed. In addition some epidermal and dermal proteins were visualized by indirect immunofluorescence using specific antibodies. Quantification of the intensity and the size of the immunostainings expressed in arbitrary units (a.u) was performed using a computer assisted image analysis system.

Results

Clinical and biophysical findings

Daily irradiation with 1 MED of SSR induced a significant increase in the clinical scores for erythema and pigmentation. Pigmentation, evaluated with a Chromameter® [2], increased

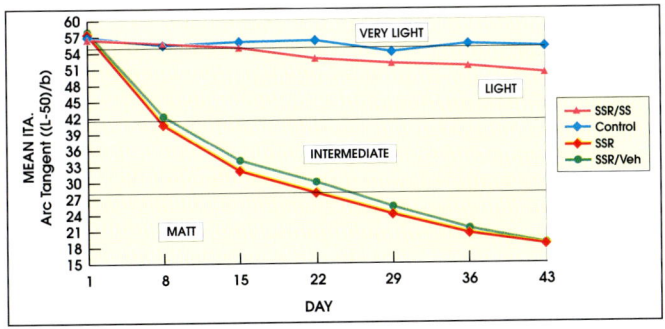

Figure 1. *Pigmentation (individual typological angle).*

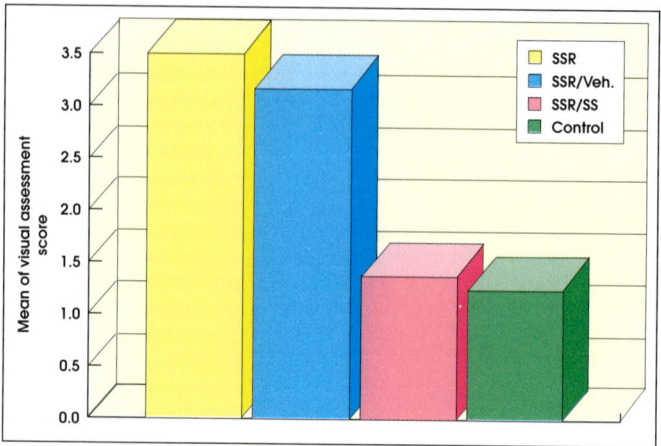

Figure 2. *Melanization (Day 43).*

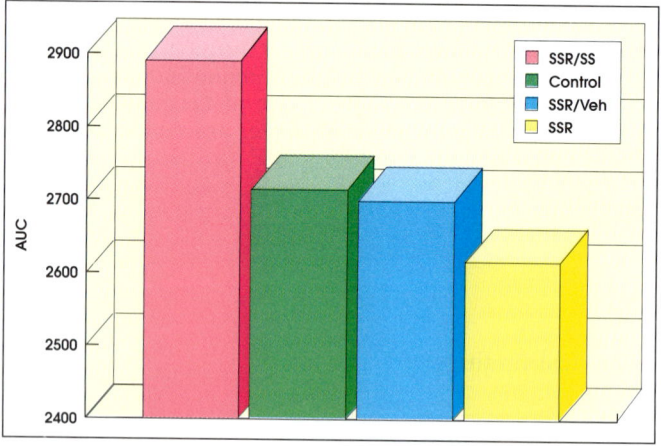

Figure 3. *Skin hydratation (AUC = Area under the curves).*

identically throughout the study in the +SSR and the +SSR/+Veh areas. In the control and +SSR/+SS sites no significant change of erythema and pigmentation was observed during the 6 week treatment. These results were supported by histological examination of melanization at day 43 using Fontana Masson staining.

The conductance, reflecting the degree of stratum corneum hydration was measured using a Dermodiag® [3]. The conductance (AUC) decreased in the +SSR site. The vehicle had a transient moisturizing effect due to its glycerin content. On the +SSR/+SS site, a high hydration level was maintained until the end of the study due to the effective protection provided by sunscreens.

Microtopography on skin replica was evaluated by visual score assessment [3]. A significant alteration of the skin microtopography was noticed after only 5 SSR exposures

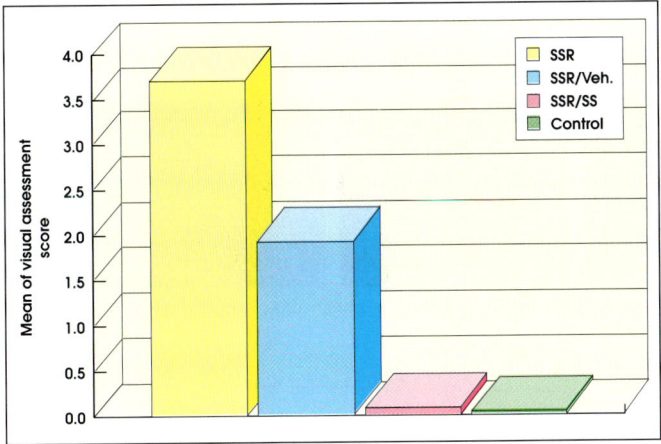

Figure 4. *Skin microtopography (Day 8).*

Table I. *Quantification of epidermal changes*				
Parameter	Control (n + 12)	+SSR (n + 12)	+SSR/Veh (n + 12)	+SSR/+SS (n + 12)
Number of stratum corneum layers	14.51 ± 0.67	20.63 ± 1.21*	19.82 ± 1.05*	14.99 ± 0.41
Stratum granulosum thickness (visual assessment)	1.00 ± 0.00	2.13 ± 0.18*	1.83 ± 0.19*	1.08 ± 0.05
Growth Fraction Ki-67 positive cells %	2.96 ± 0.72	4.38 ± 0.71	4.92 ± 0.52	3.39 ± 0.57

Data are mean ± SEM; * $p < 0.05$ composed to be Control area.

(day 8). At day 8, in the +SSR/+SS site the microtopography of the skin was maintained identical to the control site.

Histological and immunohistochemical findings

Epidermis

SSR exposures induced a significant increase in the number of stratum corneum layers and in the stratum granulosum thickness. These changes were significantly prevented by pretreatment with the daily use cream.
Cellular proliferation was investigated using a Ki-67 antibody, which reacts with a nuclear antigen expressed by cells in the G1, S, M and G2 phases of the cell cycle. The number of

A

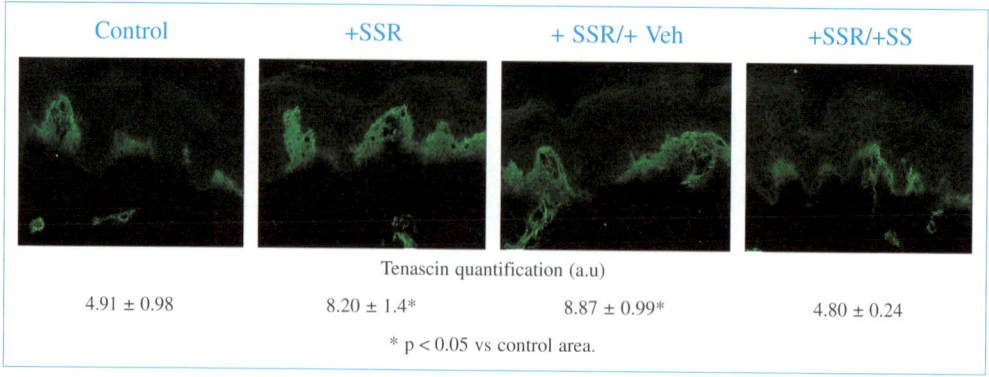

Control	+SSR	+ SSR/+ Veh	+SSR/+SS
4.91 ± 0.98	8.20 ± 1.4*	8.87 ± 0.99*	4.80 ± 0.24

Tenascin quantification (a.u)

* $p < 0.05$ vs control area.

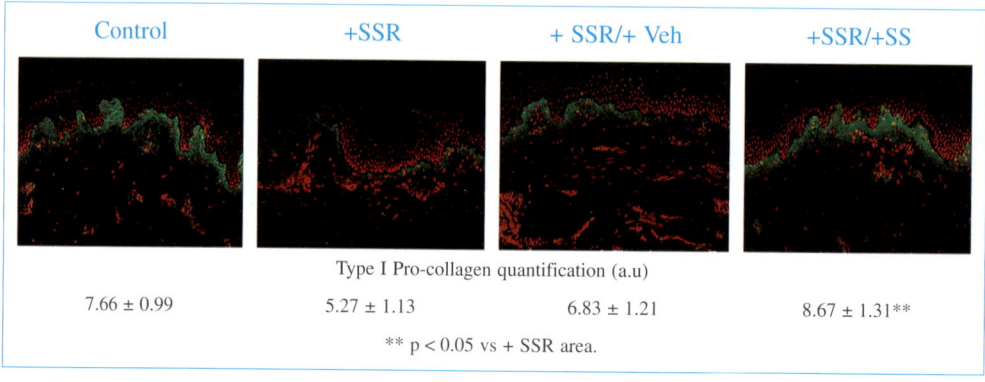

Control	+SSR	+ SSR/+ Veh	+SSR/+SS
7.66 ± 0.99	5.27 ± 1.13	6.83 ± 1.21	8.67 ± 1.31**

Type I Pro-collagen quantification (a.u)

** $p < 0.05$ vs + SSR area.

B

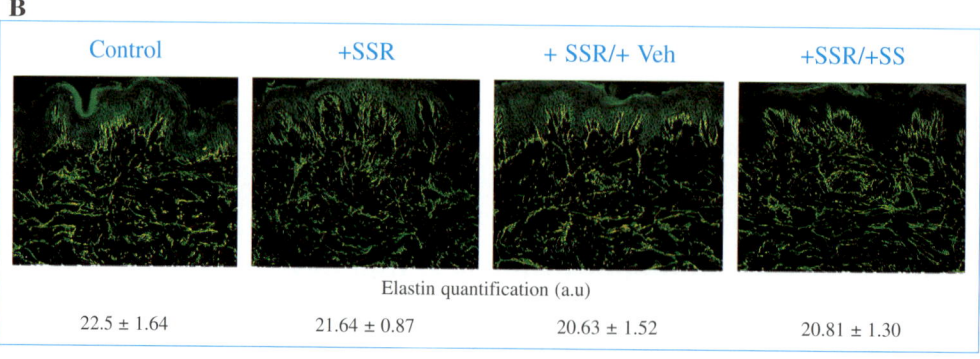

Control	+SSR	+ SSR/+ Veh	+SSR/+SS
22.5 ± 1.64	21.64 ± 0.87	20.63 ± 1.52	20.81 ± 1.30

Elastin quantification (a.u)

ki-67 positive nuclei in the epidermis were counted and expressed as a percentage of the total number of epidermal nuclei stained with propidium iodide. Pre-treatment by the daily use cream prevented cellular proliferation induced by the SSR exposures.

These results suggest that the cream tested afforded a high protection against cellular hyper-proliferation induced by SSR exposures.

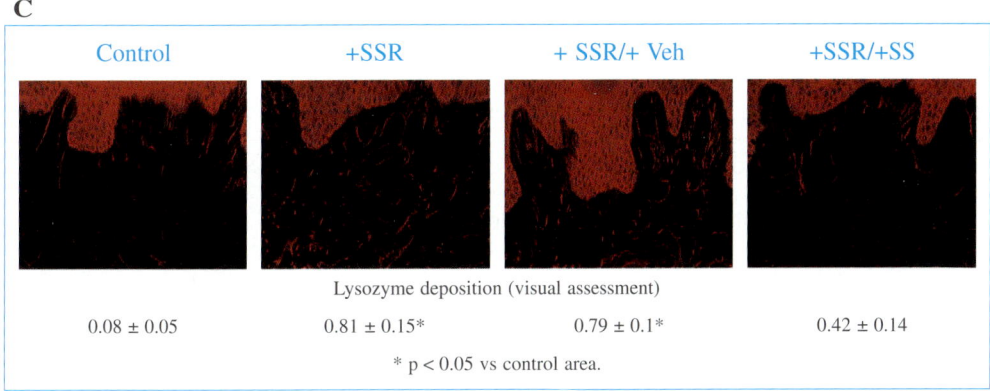

C

Control	+SSR	+ SSR/+ Veh	+SSR/+SS

Lysozyme deposition (visual assessment)

0.08 ± 0.05   0.81 ± 0.15*   0.79 ± 0.1*   0.42 ± 0.14

* $p < 0.05$ vs control area.

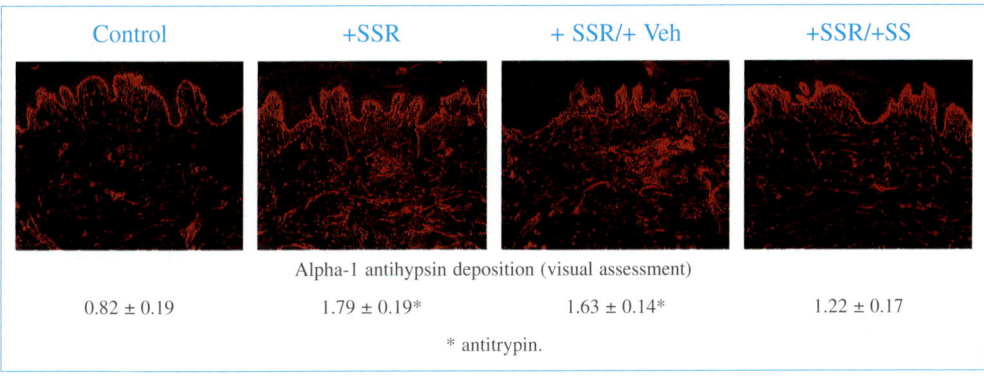

Control	+SSR	+ SSR/+ Veh	+SSR/+SS

Alpha-1 antihypsin deposition (visual assessment)

0.82 ± 0.19   1.79 ± 0.19*   1.63 ± 0.14*   1.22 ± 0.17

* antitrypin.

Dermis

No dermal inflammation was observed either at histological level or by visual assessment of the immunostaining pattern obtained after using antisera against human vimentin or factor XIII-A. A marked increase in tenascin expression (A) just below the dermal epidermal junction associated with a decrease in type I pro-collagen located at the same site were noticed after 6 weeks of SSR exposure. Pre-treatment with the daily use cream provided a very high protection against these two markers of extracellular matrix alterations related to cellular hyperproliferation for tenascin and to UVB related photoaging process for pro-collagen I [4].

A specific antibody directed against human elastin revealed an unmodified staining pattern in all exposed sites. This result supported those obtained on Luna stained sections in which no change in elastic tissue content was evidenced in all sites examined (B).

Using double immunostaining, we observed on the same sections that the dermal distribution pattern of the reaction product for lysozyme or alpha-1 antitrypsin were restricted to the elastin fiber network (C). SSR induced a significant increase in lysozyme or alpha-1antitrypsin deposition in the dermis. These deposits were prevented by pre-treatment with the daily use cream. Lysozyme or alpha-1 antitrypsin deposition on elastin fibers after SSR exposures may be considered as early events of the UVA induced elastosis process [5-6].

Conclusion

Under our experimental conditions it appears that physiological daily SSR exposures induce:
– melanogenesis,
– a decrease in skin hydration and an alteration of the skin microtopography associated with a thickening of stratum corneum and stratum granulosum,
– an enhanced expression of tenascin and a decreased expression of the type I pro-collagen (UVB marker) indicating that SSR affects cell differentiation and/or proliferation and participates in the photoaging process,
– an increased deposition of lysozyme and alpha-1 antitrypsin (UVA markers) on elastin fibers, likely contributing to solar induced elastosis process.
The protective daily use cream tested, with an effective but moderate SPF, was shown to efficiently prevent UVB and UVA induced alterations. These results are in accordance with previous studies evidencing both the need for providing an effective absorption through the entire UV spectrum and the high level of protection afforded by photostable combinations of sunscreens including the wide spectrum UVA filter Mexoryl® SX.

Acknowledgements

We thank Mrs Lombard and Verdier for histological and immunohistochemical procedures, Mrs Ressayre for statistical evaluations, Mr Chardon for technical assistance and Mr Laugier for the formulations.

References

1. Gilchrest BA. Skin aging and photoaging: an overview. *J Am Acad Dermatol* 1989; 21: 610-3.
2. Chardon A, Cretois I, Hourseau C. Skin color topology and suntanning pathways. *Int J. Cosmet Sci* 1990; 13: 191-208.
3. Lévêque JL. Non invasive measurements on photodamaged skin. In: Gilchrest B.A. (ed.). Photodamage, Cambridge, New York, 1995; 185-90.
4. Kligman LH., Akin FJ., Kligman AM. The contribution of UVA and UVB to connective tissue damage in hairless mice. *J Invest Dermatol* 1985; 84: 272-6.
5. Lavker RM, Gerberick GF, Veres DA, Irwin CJ, Kaidbey KH. Cumulative effects from repeated exposures to suberythemal doses of UVB and UVA in human skin. *J Am Acad Dermatol* 1995; 32: 53-62.
6. Park PW, Biedermann K, Mecham L, Bissett DL, Mecham RP. Lysozyme binds to elastin and protects elastin from elastase-mediated degradation. *J Invest Dermatol* 1996; 106: 1075-80.

Disparate effects of photoprotection on ultraviolet radiation-induced immunosuppression

Paul R. Bergstresser

P.R. Bergstresser: Department of Dermatology, UT Southwestern Medical Center, Dallas, Texas, USA.

To be biologically relevant, UVR must be absorbed by one or more molecules (chromophores) within target tissues. Molecules of immunologic interest have included DNA, trans-urocanic acid (*trans*-UCA), cyclic amino acids, and unsaturated membrane lipids. Under ideal circumstances, the action spectrum for a biological response is quite similar to the absorption spectrum of a candidate molecule. This method of empiric analysis is most accurate when a single and highly absorbent molecule is responsible for a specific effect, when the activation spectrum is identical to the absorption spectrum, and when the experiments are conducted *in vitro* without an interposed epidermis and stratum corneum. Unfortunately, *in vivo* systems are complicated by large numbers of candidate molecules, variable depths of candidate cells within tissues, and wave-length-dependent transmission characteristics of skin. Thus, *in vitro* systems may not include one or more relevant photoreceptors, and animal models may not substitute for human skin.

Two highly related lines of investigation have produced mouse models of immunosuppression, local and systemic. Confusion about their attributes and limitations have hindered some investigators, especially when testing the effects of photoprotection.

Local *versus* Systemic Immunosuppression: *(At the time of induction)*
Local   Hapten painted on an irradiated site induces suppression, whereas hapten painted on an unirradiated site induces conventional immunity
Systemic Hapten painted on either an irradiated or an unirradiated site induces suppression
Both   Lead to systemic suppression.

Local *versus* Systemic Immunosuppression: Implications:
Systemic immunosuppression suggests that a "factor" leaves the skin (epidermis) to operate at a distant site(s). (IL-10, TNF-alpha, and cis-UCA are candidates)

Local immunosuppression does not suggest a mechanism. (Irradiated APC, local action of a "factor", or a recruited cell have all been proposed). Genetic factors have profound effects on local immunosuppression.

Extension Animal Models of UV-induced Immonusuppression to Humans: two groups of investigators have extended to humans the studies conducted previously in rodents [1, 2].

Targets and Photoreceptors: first choice among candidate photoreceptors for UVR-induced immunosuppression has been **DNA** [3, 4]. Compelling circumstantial evidence also indicates that ***trans*-UCA**, a molecule occurring in high concentrations in the stratum corneum, is a relevant chromophore in UVR-induced immunosuppression [5]. A third hypothesis, one that has as yet received only modest attention, concerns the possibility that **unsaturated lipids** within cell membranes might serve a relevant photoreceptors for UVR-induced immunological effects [6]. Additional interesting circumstantial evidence favors the generation of **reactive oxygen species** near to or within membrane is a consequence of UVR exposure. **Irradiated LCs** alone are able to induce tolerance, as are the cells that migrate into sites of irradiation [7].

Prevention of immunosuppression with sunscreens: an interesting argument has developed in the literature concerning whether commercial sunscreens that are able to prevent UVR-induced erythema are also able to prevent immunosuppression. As this debate is reviewed, it becomes obvious that the use of irradiation equipment with differing emission spectra may have accounted for much confusion. In 1981, Lynch *et al.* [8], using unfiltered FS sunlamps in a systemic suppression model (high dose UVB, with sensitizer applied to an unirradiated site), observed that a PABA-containing sunscreen was unable to prevent the development of immunosuppression against a contact sensitizer, even though damage to skin had apparently been prevented. Some time later, Morison [9] reported that a sunscreen containing Padimate O and oxybenzone would diminished UVR-induced immunosuppression in an experimental model employing natural sunlight. But in 1989, Fisher *et al.* [10], using FS36T12-UVB-VHO lamps reported that the two sunscreens tested by Morison [9] could not prevent the development of systemic immunosuppression. Finally, Reeve *et al.* [11] reported that a sunscreen containing octyl-N-dimethyl-p-aminobenzoate (o-PABA) did not prevent the development of immunosuppression, whereas 2-ethyl-hexyl-p-methoxycinnamate (2-EHMC) did. Both sunscreens were equally effective in preventing UV-induced erythema and edema.

To reconcile these studies, and many others, it is important examine the spectral output of commonly used radiation sources, especially near 280 nm, and to compare them with natural sunlight. Roberts and Beasley [12] reported that equivalent levels of immune suppression require substantially less total energy when one uses a Kodacel-filtered radiation source (taking out most energy below 290 nm) compared with a solar simulator. This suggests that the relatively greater amounts of high energy UVB (below 290 nm) emitted even by the unfiltered FS lamps is responsible for disproportionate effects. Most importantly, sunscreen effectiveness correlated even better with SPF when using simulator radiation compared with unfiltered or filtered FS irradiation.

More recent reports have strengthened the assumption that UVR-absorbing sunscreens do protect against UVR-induced immunosuppression.

References

1. Yoshikawa T, Rae V, Bruins-Stot W, van den Berg JW, Taylor JR, Streilein JW. Susceptibility to effects of UVB radiation on induction of contact hypersensitivity as a risk factor skin cancer in man. *J Invest Dermatol* 1990; 95: 530.
2. Cooper KD, Oberhelman L, Hamilton TA, Baadsgaard O, Terhune M, LeVee G, Anderson T, Koren H. UV exposure reduces immunization rates and promotes tolerance to epicutaneous antigens in humans: relationship to dose, CD1a-DR$^+$ epidermal macrophage induction, and Langerhans cell depletion. *Proc Natl Acad Sci USA* 1992; 89: 8497.
3. Applegate LA, Ley RA, Alcalay J, Kripke ML. Identification of the molecular target for the suppression of contact hypersensitivity by ultraviolet radiation. *J Exp Med* 1989; 170: 1117.

4. Kripke ML, Cox PA, Alas LG, Yarosh DB. Pyrimidine dimers in DNA initiate systemic immunosuppression in UV-irradiated mice. *Proc Natl Acad Sci USA* 1992; 89: 7516.
5. Noonan FP, Bucana C, Sauder DN, DeFabo ED. Mechanism of systemic immune suppression by UV irradiation in vivo. II. the UV effects on number and morphology of epidermal Langerhans cells and the UV-induced suppression of contact hypersensitivity have different wavelength dependencies. *J Immunol* 1984; 132: 2408.
6. Devary Y, Rosette C, DiDonato JA, Karin M. NF-kappaB activation by ultraviolet light is not dependent on a nuclear signal. *Science* 1993; 261: 1442.
7. Cruz PD Jr, Tigelaar RE, Bergstresser PR. Langerhans cells that migrate to skin following intravenous infusion regulate the induction of contact hypersensitivity. *J Immunol* 1990; 144: 2486.
8. Lynch DH, Gurish MF, Daynes RA. Relationship between epidermal Langerhans cell density ATPase activity and the induction of contact hypersensitivity. *J Immunol* 1981; 126: 1892-7.
9. Morison WL. The effect of a sunscreen containing paraminobenyoc acid on the systemic immunologic alterations induced in mice by exposure to UVB radiation. *J Invest Dermatol* 1984; 83: 404.
10. Fisher MS, Menter JM, Willis I. Ultraviolet radiation-induced suppression of contact hypersensitivity in relation to padimate O and oxybenzone. *J Invest Dermatol* 1989; 92: 337-41.
11. Reeve VE, Bosnic M, Boehm-Wilcox C, Ley RD. Differential protection by two sunscreens from UV radiation-induced immunosuppression. *J Invest Dermatol* 1991; 97: 624-8.
12. Roberts LK, Beasley DG. Commercial sunscreen lotions prevent ultraviolet-radiation-induced immune suppression of contact hypersensitivity. *J Invest Dermatol* 1995; 105: 339-44.
13. Biestek R, Barbets RTC, Nearn MR, Halliday GM. Sunscreen protection of contact hypersensitivity responses from chronic solar-simulated ultraviolet irradiation correlates with the absorption spectrum of the sunscreen. *J Invest Dermatol* 1995; 105: 345-51.
14. Davenport V, Morris JF, Chu AC. Immunologic protection afforded by sunscreens *in vitro*. *J Invest Dermatol* 1997; 108: 859-63.
15. Elmets CA, LeVine MJ, Bickers DR. Action spectrum studies for induction of immunologic unresponsiveness to dinitrobenzene following in vivo low dose ultraviolet radiation. *Photochem Photobiol* 1985; 42: 391-7.
16. Granstein RD. Evidence that sunscreens prevent UV radiation-induced immunosuppression in humans. *Arch Dermatol* 1995; 131: 1201-4.
17. Thompson SC, Jolley D, Marks R. Reduction of solar keratoses by regular sunscreen use. *N Engl J Med* 1993; 329. 1147 51.
18. Walker SL, Young AR. Sunscreens offer the same UVB protection factors for inflammation and immunosuppression in the mouse. *J Invest Dermatol* 1997; 108: 133-8.
19. Whitemore SE, Morison WL. Prevention of UVB-induced immunosuppression in humans by a high sun protection factor sunscreen. *Arch Dermatol* 1997; 131: 1128-33.
20. Wolf P, Donawho CK, Kripke ML. Analysis of the protective effect of different sunscreens on ultraviolet radiation-induced local and systemic suppression of contact hypersensitivity and inflammatory responses in mice. *J Invest Dermatol* 1993; 100: 254.
21. Wolf P, Kripke ML. Sunscreens and immunosuppression. *J Invest Dermatol* 1996; 106: 1152-3.

Immunosuppression induced by chronic ultraviolet irradiation in humans and its prevention by sunscreens

D. Moyal

D. Moyal: L'Oréal Research, 92117 Clichy, France.

Ultraviolet radiation has been shown to induce immunosuppression. This phenomenon plays an important role in UV carcinogenesis by contributing to a decrease of the host resistance against tumor growth [1]. UV alters antigen presenting cell function by affecting directly the number, the morphology and functionality of Langerhans cells [2, 3]. It induces also the release of immunomodulating cytokines [4] and the isomerisation of urocanic acid (UCA) from trans- to cis form. The cis isomer of UCA has been reported to play an important role in the initiation of photoimmunosuppression [5, 6].

All these effects are induced by UVB and UVA and may impair the induction of local and systemic contact hypersensitivity (CHS) and delayed type reactions (DTH) to hapten applied to irradiated or unirradiated skin [7-13]. The precise mechanisms by which UV radiation induces immune suppression are still unclear.

Contradictory results have been reported on the potential of sunscreens to protect against this phenomenon [14-19].

Our research group, recently, designed human studies to examine the local and systemic effects in humans following skin exposure either to UVB + UVA radiation or to UVA alone and to evaluate the efficacy of sunscreen products. We measured the delayed type hypersensitivity (DTH) skin response and examined the efficacy of sunscreens in preventing these effects. The DTH was quantified using the recall antigens of the Multitest Kit [20-21].

For this study, volunteers were recruited after study approval by an ethical committee. Study inclusion criteria included skin type 2 or 3, age between 18 and 40 years and general good health. Exclusion criteria included conditions or medications causing immunodepression or risk of photosensitization and initial score obtained with the Multitest inferior to 5. Different groups of 10 to 12 subjects were constituted.

In a first step, the effects of exposure to UVB + UVA and to UVA alone without sunscreen were studied.

The subjects were randomised and divided into three groups. Group 1 was not exposed to UV and served as a control group which allowed to check the variability of the reaction to the Multitest in the absence of UV exposure. Group 2 was exposed to UVB + UVA, Group 3 was exposed to UVA alone.

In a second step, we compared in the Groups 4 and 5 the efficacy of two sunscreens for prevention of the immunodepression induced by UVB + UVA exposure. A control group 6 was again exposed without sunscreen.

UV radiation was applied to the centre of the back and the thorax. The exposed area on each side was approximately 600 cm^2.

Groups 2, 4, 5, 6 were exposed to the lamp which had an emission spectrum ranging from 290 to 390 nm. Group 3 was exposed to the lamp which had an UVA emission spectrum ranging from 320 to 400 nm.

The spectral power distribution was measured with a spectroradiometer Macam 3010 (Macam Scotland). The daily output was monitored with a Centra OSRAM radiometer equipped with UVB and UVA sensors.

In the groups 2 and 6 (UVA + UVB irradiated control), ten daily exposures were performed. The UV dose was progressively increased from 0.8x of the individual MED (minimal erythemal dose) to 2x of the MED. The total UVB+UVA dose was 14.5 MED per body side. The UVA dose delivered was 75 J/cm^2.

In groups 4 (UVA + UVB + sunscreen A) and 5 (UVA + UVB + sunscreen B) these UV doses were multiplied by 4.5-fold which correspond to half the Sun Protection Factor (SPF) of the sunscreens. We chose to expose the skin to UV doses that did not exceed the protective efficacy of the sunscreens against UV erythema. Thus at the last exposure the final UV dose was 9 MED which corresponds to the level of erythemal protection granted by the applied sunscreen. The total UV dose delivered was 58 individual MED and its UVA part corresponded to an average of 315 J/cm^2.

In group 3 (UVA) 12 daily exposures were performed. The UVA dose was progressively increased from 20 J/cm^2 to 50 J/cm^2. The total UVA dose received was 350 J/cm^2.

For the comparison of groups 4 and 5 (UVB + UVA) we selected two sunscreens having the same SPF 9 but with a different absorption spectra as shown in *Figure 1*. The SPF of each sunscreen was determined using the Mutzhas lamp 290-390 nm. Sunscreen A was composed of two UVB filters : 9% Octocrylene (Uvinul N539), 2% Phenylbenzimidazole Sulfonic Acid (Eusolex 232) and two UVA filters, *i.e.* one absorbing short UVA (0.7% Mexoryl® SX) and the other one absorbing long UVAs (2% Avobenzone, Parsol 1789). With such a composition the absorption spectrum of sunscreen A covered the entire UV range and had a flat spectrum profile. Sunscreen B was composed of the same UVB filters with adjusted concentrations [9% Octocrylene (Uvinul N539), 1% Phenylbenzimidazole Sulfonic Acid (Eusolex 232)] to provide the same SPF as for sunscreen A. However, the absorption spectrum of sunscreen B covered essentially the UVB range and thus its efficacy in UVA was very low. The efficacy of both sunscreens in the UVA range was assessed using the Persistent Pigment Darkening Method [22].

The UVA protection factors were respectively 9 for sunscreen A and 2 for sunscreen B.

Sunscreens A and B were applied 15 min before each exposure (approximately 2 mg/cm^2). DTH was measured by using Multitest Kits (Pasteur/Merieux). The seven test antigens were

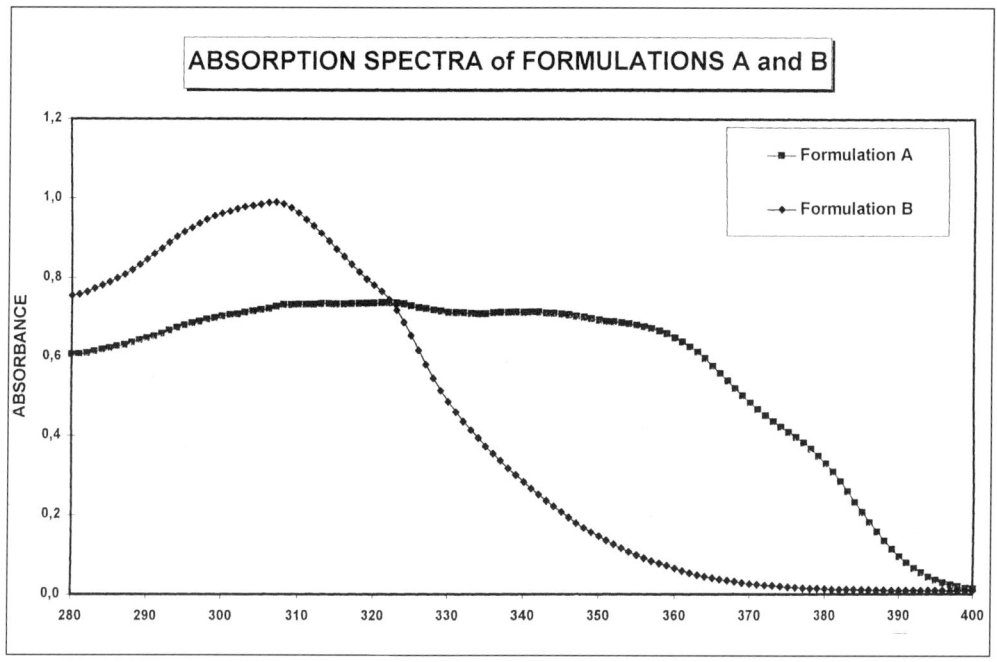

Tetanus toxoid, diphteria toxoid, *Streptococcus* antigen, tuberculin old, *Candida albicans*, *Trichophyton* and *Proteus* antigen. The negative control substance was a 70% sterile glycerin solution.

The test antigens were applied on the upper part of the back to a skin site S1 before exposure and on two additional sites 24 hours after the last UV exposure: a non-exposed skin site S2 was used for the evaluation of systemic immunodepression and an exposed skin site S3 for the assessment of both local and systemic immunodepression. Measurement of DTH test responses was made 48 hours after application of the test. The diameter of each positive test, identified as erythema accompanied by local induration, was measured in two directions with a caliper. These diameters were then averaged. To obtain the cumulative diameter (= total score) the mean diameters were added for each subject.

Differences of the DTH response after UV exposure in each group and differences of the DTH response between each group were analysed by one-way analysis of variance (SPSS software).

The results for the first part of the study are summarized in *Table I*:

No significant variation between the 3 Multitests sites was observed in the control group 1 which was not exposed to UV. A significant and similar decrease of the response to the antigens was observed in Group 2 (UVA + UVB) after exposure of the two skin sites, exposed and non-exposed. In Group 3 (UVA) a significant and equivalent decrease in the responses was also observed on the two sites. The decrease of the DTH responses observed in groups 2 and 3 which were exposed either to UVB + UVA or to UVA alone was similar on the exposed and non-exposed skin sites, the decrease was around 65%.

Table I. *Effect of the UVB + UVA and UVA irradiations DTH test responses: intergroup comparison of total score (x ± SE)*

Test site	1 Control group not-exposed	2 UVB + UVA group	3 UVA group
Pre-UV Skin site S1	10 ± 2.9	9.2 ± 3.6	8.1 ± 2.1
Post UV Skin site S2 (non exposed)	12 ± 3.4	4.3 ± 2.5[a]	3.1 ± 1.7[a]
Post UV Skin site S3 (exposed)	9.8 ± 3.3	2.9 ± 1.8[a]	2.7 ± 1.3[a]

* Significantly different from pre-UV and control group ($p < 0.05$).

The results of the second part of the study is summarised in *Table II*.

In the control group (Group 6) which was exposed to UVB + UVA without sunscreen, the decrease in the DTH response on the exposed and non-exposed skin sites was confirmed it was similar to the response observed in Group 2.

In Group 5 (UVA/UVB + sunscreen B) the decrease in the response was also observed on the two skin sites. There was no statistically significant difference between the Groups 6 and 5 on exposed and non-exposed skin sites.

In Group 4 (UVA/UVB + sunscreen A) the DTH response was slightly decreased (– 27%) on the exposed site and unchanged on the non-exposed site.

In the first part of the study we have shown that the response to the DTH tests was statisti-

Table II. *Efficacy of two sunscreens DTH test responses: intergroup comparison of total score (x ± SE)*

Test site	6 Control group exposed without sunscreen	4 Exposed with sunscreen A	5 Exposed with sunscreen B
Pre-UV Skin site S1	13.8 ± 4.5	13.1 ± 2.9	13.3 ± 3.3
Post UV Skin site S2 (non exposed)	4.5 ± 2.3[a]	11.5 ± 2.4[b]	6.3 ± 1.9[a]
Post UV Skin site S3 (exposed)	3.5 ± 2[a]	9.2 ± 1.9[ab]	4.6 ± 2.2[a]

[a] Significantly different from pre-UV ($p < 0.05$) for each group.
[b] Significantly different from Group 6 and Group 5 ($p < 0.05$) for the same skin site.

cally significantly reduced by exposure to UVB + UVA or UVA radiation alone. In both cases, the immune response was lower both locally and systemicaly. The degree of suppression was similar for UVA/UVB and UVA alone.

The absence of a decrease in immune response at non-exposed sites in Group 4 (UVA/UVB + sunscreen A) suggests that a application of this sunscreen prevents the systemic immunodepression. The efficacy of this filter is confirmed by the observed decrease (− 27%) on the exposed site which was less marked than the effect observed in the control group. This suggests that the sunscreen A also reduces the local immune depression.

Given that the UVB sunscreen failed to provide local and systemic immunoprotection against UVA/UVB, the results confirm that UVA significantly contribute to the induction of photoimmunodepression.

Comparing UVB- and UVA/UVB-sunscreens with similar SPF, it appears that the sunscreen which provides additional protection in the UVA range reduces the local UV induced immunodepression and prevents the systemic effects.

Furthermore, the results of this study suggest that SPF which is based on acute erythema is not suitable as an indicator for the protective efficacy of sunscreens against photoimmunodepression.

In a following study, we evaluate, in humans volunteers, under real sun exposure conditions, the efficacy of a new broadspectrum sunscreen product in preventing loss of DTH response.

DTH tests were performed before and after sun exposure of the upper part of the back. A non exposed area (forearm) was used as control. Prior to sun exposures 14 subjects were treated with the new sunscreen formula. This sunscreen has both a very high sun (SPF > 60) and UVA (UVAPF = 28), Persistent Pigment Darkening method (PPD) protection factors. Moreover, the following UV filtering system: UVB filter (Octocrylene), UVA filters (Mexoryl® SX, Mexoryl® XL, Avobenzone), TiO_2 allows the formula to be photostable.

The volunteers were sun exposed during 6 days. They received a total UV dose equivalent to 64 minimal erythemal dose (MED) and 400 J/cm^2 of UVA.

Compared to the DTH response we obtained before sun exposure, we did not detect any significant changes in the immune response on the exposed site (back) and on the non-exposed site (forearm).

We have demonstrated that, under intensive sunlight exposure, the use of a highly protective UVB + UVA sunscreen can prevent from photo-immunosuppression. This is of particular importance if we consider the possible link between immunosuppression and skin cancers developments.

Our different studies based on repeated exposures simulate the real-life situation and clearly demonstrate the need for sunproducts protecting throughout the entire UV spectrum and offering high SPF as well as high UVA-PF to afford immunoprotection.

References

1. Nishigori C, Yarosh DB, Donawho C, et al. The immune system in ultraviolet carcinogenesis. *J Invest Dermatol Symp Proc* 1996: 143-6
2. Ullrich SE. Modulation of immunity by ultraviolet radiation: key effects on antigen presentation. *J Invest Dermatol* 1995; 105: 30S-6S.
3. Cooper KD, Fox P, Neises G, et al. Effects of ultraviolet radiation on human epidermal cell alloantigen presentation: initial depression of Langerhans cell-dependant function is followed by the appearance of T6DR+ cells that enhance epidermal alloantigen presentation. *J Immunol* 1985; 134: 129-37.
4. Kim TY, Kripke ML, Ullrich SE. Immunodepression by factors released from UV-irradiated epidermal cells : selective effects on the generation of contact and delayed hypersensitivity after exposure to UVA or UVB radiation. *J Invest Dermatol* 1990; 94: 26-32.
5. De Fabo EC, Noonan FP. Mechanism of immunosupression by UV irradiation *in vivo:* evidence for the existence of a unique photoreceptors in the skin and its role in photoimmunology. *J Exp Med* 1983; 157: 84-98.
6. Gibbs NK, Norval M, Traynor NJ, Wolf M, Johnson BA, Crosby J. Action spectra for the trans to cis photoisomerization of urocanic acid *in vitro* and in mouse skin. *Photochem Photobiol* 1993; 57: 584-90.
7. Levee GJ, Oberhelman L, Anderson T, Koren H, Cooper KD. UVAII exposure of human skin results in decreased immunization capacity, increased induction of tolerance and a unique pattern of epidermal antigen-presenting cell alteration. *Photochem Photobiol* 1997; 65: 622-9.
8. Streilein JW, Bergstresser PR. Genetic basis of ultraviolet-B effects on contact hypersentivity. *Immunogenetics* 1988; 27: 252-8.
9. Cooper KD, Oberhelman L, Hamilton TA, Baadsgaard O, Terhune M, Levee G, Anderson T, Koren H. UV exposure reduces immunization rates and promotes tolerance to epicutaneous antigens in humans -relationship to dose, CD1a-DR + epidermal macrophage induction, and Langerhans cell depletion. *Proc Natl Acad Sci USA* 1992; 89: 8497-501.
10. Morison WL, Pike RA, Kripke ML. Effect on sunlight and its component wavebands on contact hypersensitivity in mice and guinea-pig. *Photodermatol* 1985; 2: 195-204.
11. Cooper KD. Effects of UV radiation from artificial light sources on the human immune system. *Photochem Photobiol* 1995; 61: 231-5.
12. Yoshikawa T, Rae V, Bruins-Hot W, Vander Berg JW, Taylor JR, Streilein JW. Susceptibility to effects of UVB radiation on induction of contact hypersensitivity as a risk factor for skin cancer in humans. *J Invest Dermatol* 1990; 95: 530-6.
13. Schwartz. Effects of UVA light on the immune system. A settled issue? *Eur J Dermatol* 1996; 6: 227-8.
14. Van Praag MCG, Out-Luyting C, Claas FHJ, Vermeer BJ, Mommaas AM. Effect of topical sunscreens on the UV-radiation induced suppression of the alloactivating capacity in human skin *in vivo*. *J Invest Dermatol* 1991; 97: 629-33.
15. Wolf P, Kripke ML. Sunscreens and immunity. *Skin cancer* 1993; 8: 33-40.
16. Wolf P, Donawho CK, Kripke ML. Analysis of the protective effect of different sunscreens on ultraviolet radiation induced local and systemic suppression of contact hypersensitivity and inflammatory responses in mice. *J Invest Dermatol* 1993; 100: 254-9.
17. Whitmore SE, Morison WL. Prevention of UVB induced immunosuppression in humans by a high sun protection factor sunscreen. *Arch Dermatol* 1995; 131: 1128-33.
18. Bestak R, Barnetson RSC, Nearn MR, Halliday GM. Sunscreen protection of contact hypersensitivity. Responses from chronic solar simulated ultraviolet irradiation correlates with the absorption spectrum of the sunscreen. *J Invest Dermatol* 1995; 105: 345-51.
19. Roberts LK, Beasley DG. Commercial sunscreen lotions prevent ultraviolet radiation induced immunosuppression of contact hypersensitivity. *J Invest Dermatol* 1995; 105: 339-44.

20. Hersey P, Mac Donald DM, Burns C, Schibeci S, *et al*. Analysis of the effect of a sunscreen agent on the suppression of Natural Killer Cell activity induced in human subjects by radiation from solarium lamps. *J Invest Dermatol* 1987; 88: 271-6.
21. Fuller CJ, Faulkner H, Bendich A, Parker RS, Roe DA. Effect of β carotene supplementation on photosuppression of delayed type hypersensitivity in normal young men. *Am J Clin Nutr* 1992; 56: 684-90.
22. Chardon A, Moyal D, Hourseau C. Persistent pigment darkening response as a method for evaluation of ultraviolet A protection assays. In *Sunscreens, 2nd edition* (Edited by N.J. Lowe, Nadim A. Shaath, Madhu A. Pathak) Marcel Dekker, Inc. New-York, Basel, Hong-Kong 1997: 559-82.

Photoprotection and photo-immunosuppression in man

L. Meunier

L. Meunier: Department of Dermatology-Allergology-Photobiology, St-Éloi Hospital, University of Montpellier, Montpellier, France.

The immune system plays an important role in ultraviolet (UV) carcinogenesis by contributing to host resistance against tumor growth, and individuals sensitive to UVB-induced immunosuppression are at increased risk for the development of skin cancer. Thus, both UV-induced DNA alterations as well as immune regulation are important for cutaneous carcinogenesis. UV radiation (UVR) alters antigen-presenting cell function directly by affecting epidermal Langerhans cells (LC) or indirectly by inducing keratinocytes to release immunomodulatory cytokines. Chemical sunscreens (SS) have been shown to prevent UV-induced sunburn, actinic keratosis, photoageing, and DNA damage. However, there are conflicting reports regarding the efficacy of SS in preventing UV-induced immunosuppression [1]. Results of these reports should be viewed with caution because FS-40 sunlamps, which emit shorter wavelengths of UV radiation than solar radiation were employed. Furthermore the sun protection factor (SPF) of the tested SS has to comply with the dose and the type of UVR that is utilized in the experimental design. It is therefore difficult to extrapolate to humans results of studies performed on animals under various experimental conditions. In humans, few studies have been performed to assess the ability of SS to prevent UV-induced immunosuppression. The mixed-lymphocyte reaction (MLR) was first used to test the protective capacity of several sunscreens as UVB exposure of stimulator cells (lymphocytes) resulted in a decreased alloactivating capacity. Tested sunscreens partly abrogated the UV-induced decrease of the immune response [2]. By using the mixed epidermal cell-lymphocyte reaction (MECLR) system, local applications of sunscreens on a limited skin area did not prevent the UV-induced suppression of the alloactivating capacity after 4 weeks of either UVB or PUVA therapy [3]. Thus, people protected from sunburn by sunscreens may be exposed to UV for a long period of time, and thereby subject themselves to its immunosuppressive action. By contrast, the same sunscreen prevented the increase of the MECLR and the influx of $CD36^+DR^+$ cells that was observed after a short-term (4 days) erythemagenic UVB exposure [4] indicating that the protective effect of SS is critically dependent on the UV protocol used. UV-exposure of human skin explants with and without prior application of a cream allows investigation of the impairment of the MECLR by UV radiation and the immune protection afforded by several SS [5]. By using the model, SS tested protected beyond their *in vitro* SPF values. Pretreatment of skin with cosmetic preparations containing photoprotective agents (SPF 15) provided complete protection against sunburn cell formation and LC damage in individuals whose skin was exposed to a UVB dose corresponding to 1.5 MED each day for 4 consecutive days [6]. Sunscreen use is protective against a short-term sun exposure but does not prevent the reduction in the number of LC induced by chronic sun exposure [7]. Cutaneous exposure to UVB radiation impairs the induction of contact hypersensitivity (CHS) to hapten applied on the irradiated skin surface in humans [8]. Therefore the experimental model of CHS may be proposed to explore the *in vivo* relationships between UV and cutaneous immunity although various factors such as UV doses, timing of sensitization after irradiation, hapten concentration, age, sex and genetic background of the responder determine the strength of the reactions. Whitmore and Morison [9] demonstrated that application of a SS with over ninefold greater protection than that needed to prevent erythema, prior to localized UVB radiation, prevents localized UVB-induced suppression of CHS after a daily 3 MED UVB exposure for 3 consecutive days. Recently, we showed that a SPF 15 SS with high UVA protection could prevent the reduction of CHS responses cause by an acute solar-simulated UV exposure [10]. We utilized multiple control groups to ensure that the sunscreen preparation did not modify by itself, the induction of CHS and to determine the threshold of allergic responses with a statistically significant number of subjects. To assess the protective effect of SS on UV-induced inhibition of the immune effector mechanisms, Damian *et al.* [11] demonstrated that broad-spectrum SS provided greater protection against UV-induced suppression of the CHS response to nickel in nickel-allergic subjects. Moyal *et al.* [12] examined the effects of UVR on delayed-type hypersensitivity and showed that under UVB + UVA exposure, a UVB SS failed to provide local and systemic immunoprotection whereas a SS having the same SPF with an adequate UVA protection prevented the systemic effects. The ability of SS to provide immunoprotection is critically dependent on the UV treatment. The light source is important and should correspond to that used to establish the SS formulation. Recent results emphasize the need for adequate UVA protection.

References

1. Wolf P, Kripke ML. Sunscreens and immunity. *Skin Cancer* 1993; 8: 33-40.
2. Mommaas AM, van Praag MCG, Bavinck JNB, Out-Luiting C, Vermeer BJ, Claas FHJ. Analysis of the protective effect of topical sunscreens on the UVB-radiation-induced suppression of the mixed-lymphocyte reaction. *J Invest Dermatol* 1990; 95: 313-6.
3. van Praag MCG, Out-Luyting C, Claas FHJ, Vermeer B, Mommaas AM. Effect of topical sunscreens on the UV-radiation-induced suppression of the alloactivating capicity in human skin *in vivo*. *J Invest Dermatol* 1991; 97: 629-33.
4. Hurks HM, van der Molen RG, Out-Luiting C, Vermeer BJ, Claas FH, Mommaas AM. Differential effects of sunscreens on UVB-induced immunomodulation in humans. *J Invest Dermatol* 1997; 109: 699-703.
5. Davenport V, Morris JF, Chu AC. Immunologic protection afforded by sunscreens *in vitro*. *J Invest Dermatol* 1997; 108: 859-63.
6. Elmets CA, Vargas A, Oresajo C. Photoprotective effects of sunscreens in cosmetics on sunburn and Langerhans cell photodamage. *Photodermal Photoimmunol Photomed* 1992; 9: 113-20.
7. Neale R, Russel A, Muller HK, Green A. Sun exposure, sunscreens and their effects on epidermal Langerhans cells. *Photochem Photobiol* 1997; 66: 260-4.
8. Cooper KD, Oberhelman L, Hamilton TA, Baadsgaard O, Terhune M, Levee G, Anderson T, Koren H. UV exposure reduces immunization rates and promotes tolerance to epicutaneous antigens in humans: relationship to dose, CD1a-DR+ epidermal macrophage induction, and Langerhans cell depletion. *Proc Nat Acad Sci USA* 1992; 89: 8497-501.
9. Whitmore SE, Morison WL. Prevention of UVB-induced immunosuppression in humans by a sun protection factor sunscreen. *Arch Dermatol* 1995; 131: 1128-33.
10. Serre I, Cano JP, Picot MC, Meynadier J, Meunier L. Immunosuppression induce by acute solar-simulated ultraviolet exposure in humans: prevention by a sunscreen with a sun protection factor of 15 and high UVA protection. *J Am Acad Dermatol* 1997; 37: 187-94.

11. Damian DL, Halliday GM, Barnetson RSC. Broad-spectrum sunscreens provide greater protection against ultraviolet-radiation-induced suppression of contact hypersensitivity to a recall antigen in humans. *J Invest Dermatol* 1997; 109: 146-51.
12. Moyal D, Courbière C, Le Corre Y, de Lacharrière O, Hourseau C. Immunosuppression induced by chronic solar-simulated irradiations in humans and its prevention by sunscreens. *Eur J Dermatol* 1997; 7: 223-5.

Influence of high protective sunscreens on the photoisomerization of urocanic acid in human skin

P. Krien, D. Moyal, A. Rougier

P. Krien: Life Sciences, L'Oréal Advanced Research Laboratories, Clichy, France.
D. Moyal: L'Oréal, Applied Research and Development, Clichy, France.
A. Rougier: La Roche-Posay, Pharmaceutical Laboratories, Courbevoie, France.

Taking into account the following properties of urocanic acid:
– production of *trans*- urocanic acid (UCA) in the skin is due to the enzymatic deamination of histidine [1] ;
– under UVB (290-320 nm) and UVA (320-400 nm) exposure *trans*- to *cis*-UCA and *cis*- to *trans*-UCA conversions occur [2, 3] ;
– UCA photoisomerization is independent of skin type. This indicates that UCA photoisomerization and erythema are independent processes [4] ;
– *cis*-UCA can be involved in some immunosuppressive mechanisms [5] ;
we have used the photoproduction of *cis*-UCA in human skin exposed to UVB+A or UVA radiation as a physiological dosimeter in order to compare the protection efficiency of some sunscreens having different Sun Protection Factor (SPF) and UVA Protection Factor (UVAPF).

Materials and methods

Subjects

Fifteen healthy informed volunteers with skin type II participated in the study. Only volunters non exposed to sunlight or solar simulator since a minimum of 3 months were selected.

UV sources

A Supersun Mutzhas lamp with an emission spectrum between 290-390 nm was used as UVB+A source and with an emission spectrum in the 320-400 nm range as UVA source. Dosimetric measurements were performed using a Centra Osram uvmeter.

Sunscreens

Three commercial sunscreens were evaluated in the study.
– Sunscreen A * (SPF 60 and UVA PF** 12),
– Sunscreen D (SPF > 60 and UVA PF 3),
– Sunscreen M (SPF 8 and UVA PF 2).

* Anthelios L – La Roche-Posay, Laboratoire Pharmaceutique – France.
** Protection factor based on the Persistent Pigment Darkening (PPD) reaction [6].
mPF spectra were obtained *in vitro* after application of 1 mg/cm^2 of sunscreen on a quartz plate. First measurements were performed 15 min after application of the sunscreen on the plate and before UV exposure. Second measurements were performed after 1 hour UV exposure (Suntest lamp, dose ~ 18 J/cm^2 UVB + UVA).

Sunscreens A and M were not influenced by UV exposure whereas protection efficiency of sunscreen D decreased significantly both in the UVB and UVA ranges.

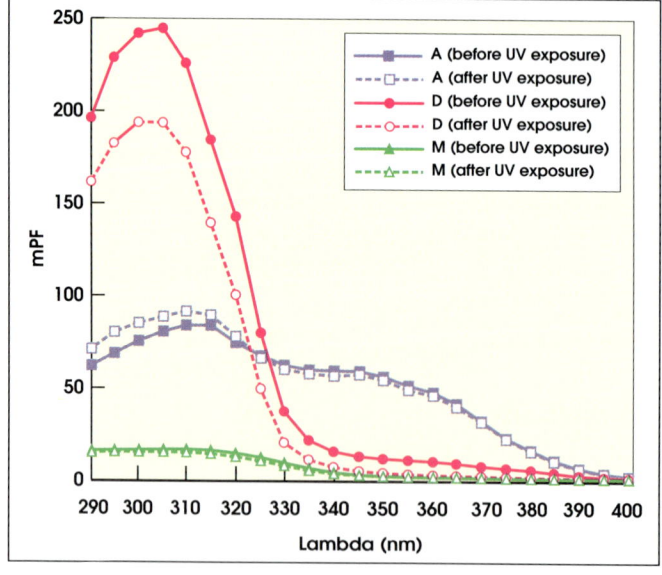

Figure 1. *Monochromatic protection factor spectra of the 3 sunscreens tested before and after UV exposure.*

Study design

Two mg/cm² of each sunscreen were applied onto a defined area of the back 15 min before a single UVB+A (290-390 nm) or UVA (320-400 nm) exposure.

At the end of exposure, 6 successive tape strippings (4 cm² area) were performed on each area using adhesive disks (Haas, Sumoreau, France). *trans-* and *cis-*UCA in each strip were quantified by HPLC [4].

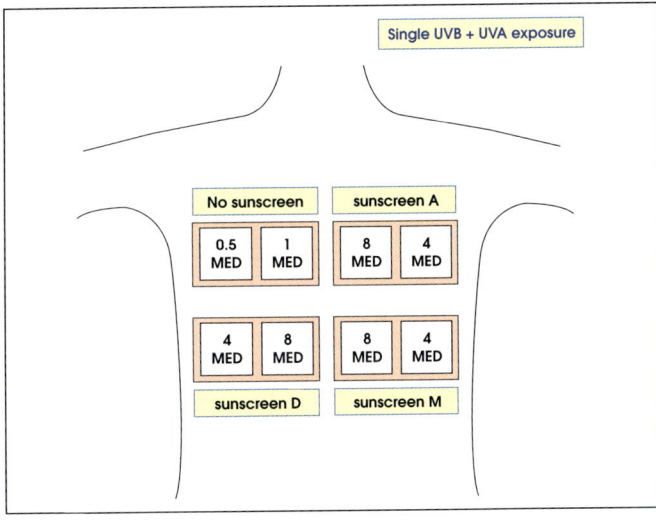

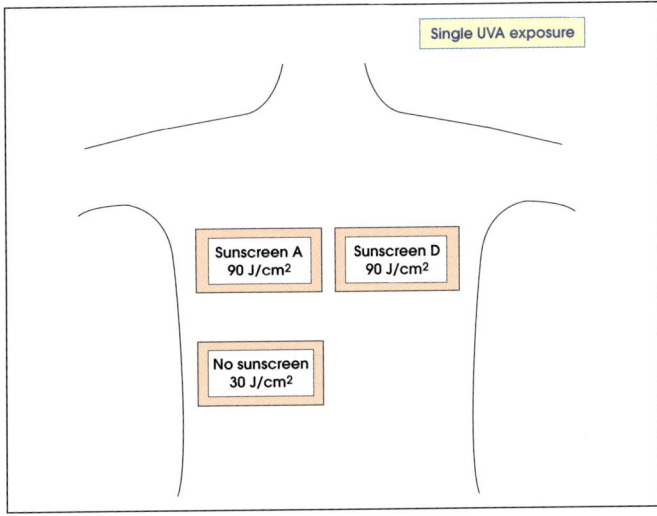

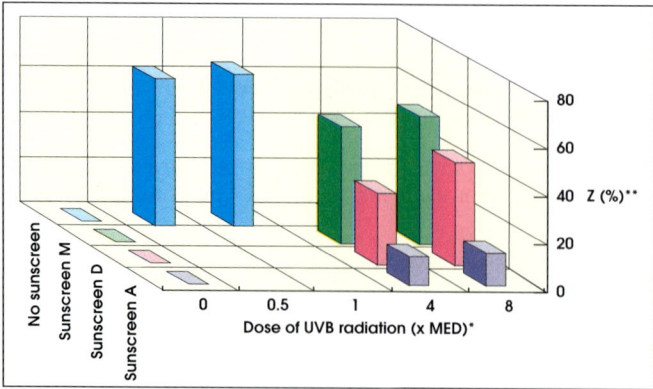

Figure 2. *Relative amount of cis-UCA after a single UVB + UVA exposure:*
* *(1 MED = 250 mJ/cm^2 UVB + 4.6 J/cm^2 UVA),*
** *Z (%) = percentage of UCA present under the cis form.*

Effects of UVA exposure

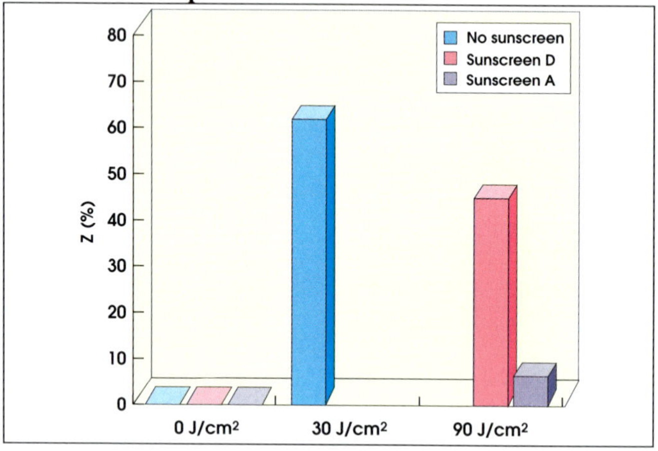

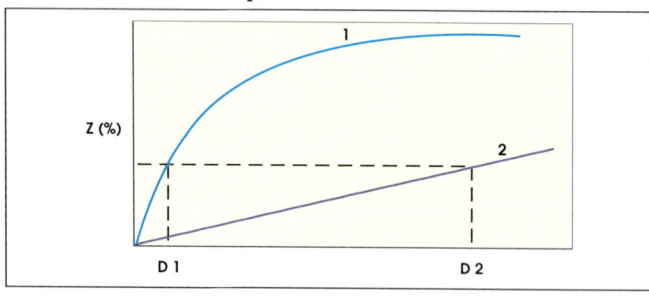

Figure 3. *Relative amount of cis-UCA after a single UVA exposure.*

Prevention of *cis*-UCA production

Figure 4. *Influence of the dose on the production of cis-UCA. Z (%) represents the percentage of cis-UCA present at a given irradiation dose. Indices « 1 » and « 2 » correspond to non protected and sunscreen protected areas, respectively.*

Table I. **Comparison of cis-UCA protection factor SFP and UVA PF of the sunscreens tested**

Sunscreen	UVA PF	cis-UCA protection factor	SPF
A	12	250	60
D	3	40	> 60
M	2	20	8

Results and discussion

Effects of UVB + A exposure
Sunscreen A (SPF 60, UVA PF 12) is more efficient in preventing cis-UCA formation than sunscreen D (SPF > 60, UVA PF 3) and sunscreen M (SPF 8, UVA PF 2). Such an observation confirms that:
– UVA are highly effective in producing cis-UCA.
– UCA photoisomerization and erythema are independent processes.

It results from this that the protective efficacy of a sunscreen should not be described using a single erythemal protection factor (SPF) [7] but requires information about its effectiveness in the UVA range.

This experiment confirmed the high contribution of the UVA in the production of cis-UCA. Only the highly protective broad-spectrum sunscreen A decreased significantly cis-UCA production induced by a single UVA exposure.
Prevention of *cis*-UCA production can be assessed by using a « *cis*-UCA protection factor » such as: *cis*-UCA protection factor = D2 / D1.
These values clearly indicate that a significant decrease in the *cis*-UCA formation requires the use of broad-spectrum (UVB plus UVA), highly protective sunscreens.
Because there is no direct relationship between UCA photoisomerization process and erythema, we suggest this reaction may be used as a complementary parameter in the assessment of the UV protection provided by sunscreens.
As a consequence of the influence of UVA in producing cis-UCA, a link between the UVA Protection Factor and the cis-UCA Protection Factor seems to be observed.

Conclusion

A significant decrease in the cis-UCA production rate can be obtained only using potent sunscreen providing high UVB and UVA protection.

Such enhanced protection was provided by an optimised photostable filtering system covering the entire UV spectrum (UVB + UVA), composed of Mexoryl® SX, PARSOL® 1789, Eusolex® 6300 and TiO_2.

Furthermore, this study clearly indicates that the protection efficiency of a sunscreen cannot be described with a single UV protection factor but requires information about its effectiveness both in the UVB and in the UVA ranges.

Acknowledgements

It is a pleasure for the authors to thank: J. Bover, F. Canivet, G. Crosnier, G. Desbois, M. Jolimay, C. Mazilier for their active and efficient collaboration in this study.

References

1. Scott IR. Biochem J. 1981; 194: 829-38
2. Schwarz W, Shell H, Hüttinger G, Wasmeier H, Diepgen T. *Photodermatology* 1987; 6: 269-71.
3. Norval M, Simpson TJ, Bardshiri E, Crosby J. *Photodermatology* 1989; 6: 142-5.
4. Krien P, Moyal D. Photochem. *Photobiol* 1994; 60: 280-7.
5. Norval M, Gibbs NK & Gilmour J. Photochem. *Photobiol* 1995; 62: 209-17.
6. Chardon A, Moyal D, Hourseau C. « Sunscreens, Development, Evaluation, and regulatory aspects » Marcel Dekker, *Inc.* 1977; 559-82.
7. van Praag MCG, Luyting CO, Claas FHJ, Vermeer BJ, Mommaas AM. *J Invest Dermatol* 1991; 97: 629-33.

The use of a reconstructed epidermis in the evaluation of protective effect of sunscreens against lipoperoxidation induced by UVA

C. Cohen, R. Roguet, M. Cottin, M.H. Grandidier, E. Popovic,
J. Leclaire, A. Rougier

C. Cohen, R. Roguet, M. Cottin, M.H. Grandidier, E. Popovic, J. Leclaire: Life Sciences, L'Oréal Advanced Research Laboratories, Aulnay-sous-Bois, France.
A. Rougier: La Roche-Posay Pharmaceutical Laboratories, Courbevoie, France.

The skin is permanently exposed to environmental factors including chemical substances and physical agents such as UV irradiation. Besides, there is increasing evidence that UVA can contribute to cutaneous photodamages including skin aging, inflammatory disorders and cancerization. Among the different mechanisms involved in these adverse effects of UVA, it is well established that the oxigenated free radicals produced play a determinent role.

Today, skin and epidermal equivalents represent the most promising biological models to assess cutaneous irritancy *in vitro*. Their advantage over culture of keratinocyte in monolayer is the presence of a fully differentiated horny layer similar, if not identical, to the *in vivo stratum corneum*. The presence of this cornified layer allows testing of lipophilic molecules as well as finished products.

The aim of the present study was to determine whether reconstructed skin or epidermis could constitute valuable *in vitro* models for the measurment of the preventive effect of sunscreen products against lipoperoxidation induced by UVA.

Materials and methods

Reconstructed human epidermis Episkin

Episkin was provided by Imedex-Saduc (Chaponost, France) as a kit containing 12 units of epidermis. One unit consists of collagen matrix (types I and III) fixed at the bottom of a plastic chamber, coated with a thin layer of collagen IV. Human adult keratinocytes seeded on this dermal substitute were grown submerged for 3 days in the medium (DMEM/HAM

F12 (3:1) + 10% fetal calf serum) and exposed at the air-liquid interface for 10 days to give rise to a fully differentiated epidermis. Like the living human epidermis, Episkin presents a *stratum corneum* which is the ultimate state of differentiation of the epidermal cells.

UVA radiation source

The UVA source was a 1,000 W solar simulator Oriel (model 68820) presenting a 102 x 102 mm size beam. In combination with additionnal filters: Oriel n° 81050 (= Schott UG11-1 mm) and Oriel n° 81019 (= Schott WG 335-3 mm) it was emitting in the 320-400 range with a maximum at 360 nm. The irradiance (13 mW/cm^2/sec) was monitored with a Osram Centra UV-meter.

Tested formulas

4 sunscreen formulas were evaluated for their ability to protect the reconstructed epidermis from UVA (50 J/cm^2) induced lipoperoxidation. Their qualitative compositions in terms of UV protective ingredients are reported in *Table I*.

Table I.

		Composition							
		UVB filters				UVA filters		Nano pigments	
		EUSOLEX® 232	UVINUL® T150	PARSOL® MCX	EUSOLEX® 6300	PARSOL® 1789	MEXORYL®SX	TIO$_2$	ZnO
Formulas	A*				●	●	●	●	
	B**				●	●	●	●	
	C	○	○	○		○		○	
	D							○	○

* Anthelios T, La Roche-Posay Pharmaceutical Laboratories.
** Anthelios L, La Roche-Posay Pharmaceutical Laboratories.

Treatment of the Episkin samples

2 mg/cm^2 of each formula were applied in duplicate on the Episkin surfaces. The wells were incubated for one hour at 37° C/5% CO$_2$ before irradiation. The epidermal equivalents were tested for lipoperoxidation immediatly after UVA exposure without rinsing out the formula (a complete removing is impossible). Eighteen hours after irradiation, the Episkin epithelia were tested for cell viability using the MTT conversion test described by Mosmann (1983) and 2 ml of underlying culture media were collected for IL1α determinations (ELISA).

Lipoperoxide production

Epidermal equivalents were crushed and extracted in isopropanol. Lipid peroxides were then measured using the K-Assay LPO-CC (KAMIYA Biomedical Company). Cumene hydroperoxide was used to generate standard curves to calibrate this very sensitive colorimetric test.

Results

UVA induced lipoperoxidation and cytotoxicity

As shown in *Figure 1*, there exists a linear relationship between the dose of UVA (0 to 100 J/cm^2) and the amount of lipoperoxides produced by the epidermis. When cells were depleted in glutathion content using the glutathion synthase inhibitor: buthionine sulfoximine (BSO),

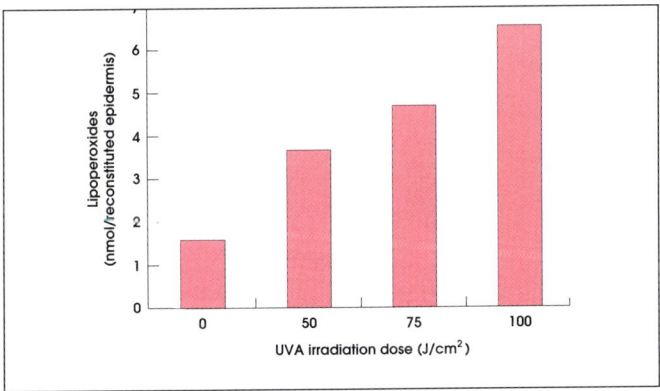

Figure 1. *UVA irradiation dose effect on lipoperoxidation in reconstructed epidermis.*

we observed an increase in lipoperoxide production *(Figure 2)* coming with an early apparition of UVA induced cellular damage *(Figure 3a)*. As a matter of fact, a non cytotoxic UVA dose of 50 J/cm^2 resulted in a complete killing of the epidermal cells *(Figure 3a)*. This confirms that glutathion cellular level is essential in protecting and detoxifying the epidermis from the lipoperoxides induced by UVA irradiation. In addition UVA doses ranking from 20 to 60 J/cm^2 led to the release of the cytokine IL1α in a dose-dependent manner, whereas they were not effective in inducing the release of this mediator under normal conditions *(Figure 3b)*. Thus when epidermal cells present lower defense (glutathion content) against oxidative stress, solar UVA light results in greater lipoperoxide production coming with greater epidermal damage.

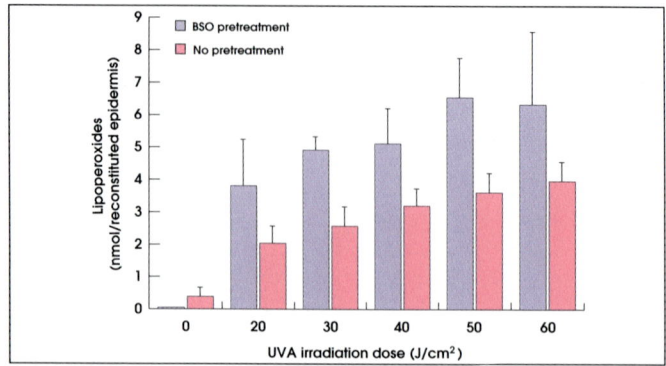

Figure 2. *UVA induced lipoperoxidation in normal and glutathion depleted reconstructed epidermis.*

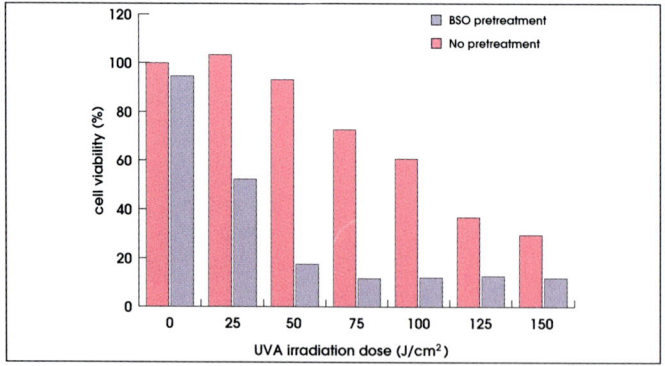

Figure 3a. *Effect of epidermal depletion in glutathion UVA induced cytotoxicity.*

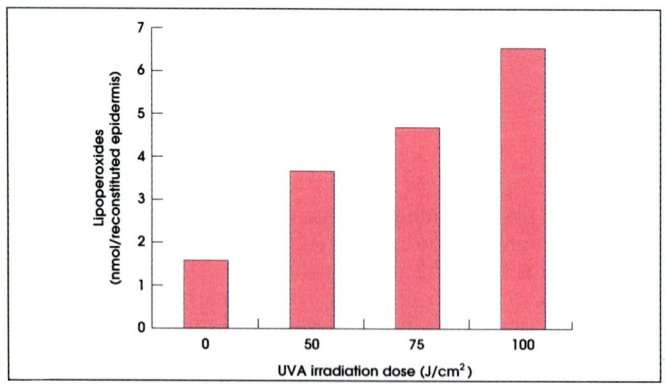

Figure 3b. *Effect of epidermal depletion in glutathion on UVA induced IL1α production.*

Efficacy of sunscreen formulas against UVA induced lipoperoxidation

This study was performed using a non cytotoxic UVA exposure dose (50 J/cm^2) without BSO pretreatment. The protective effect against lipid peroxidation of different sunscreen formulas was investigated. As shown in *Figure 4*, treating the reconstructed epidermis with formula A or B resulted in a significant reduction (50%) of the lipoperoxide production compared to their respective placebo. Placebo of formulas C and D being not available, such an evaluation on formulas C and D was not possible. *Figure 5* clearly shows that the 4 formulas investigated were extremely different with regards to their ability to protect the epidermis from an *in situ* production of lipoperoxides. As compared to the amount of lipoper-oxides produced by non protected irradiated epidermis, a striking lipoperoxide formation was induced by UVA when using formula C. On the contrary, no significant raise in lipoperoxides was found when using formulas B and D. A significant reduction was only observed when protection was afforded by formula A. Thus using in vitro human epidermis we acquired better understanding on the protective effect of sunscreens.

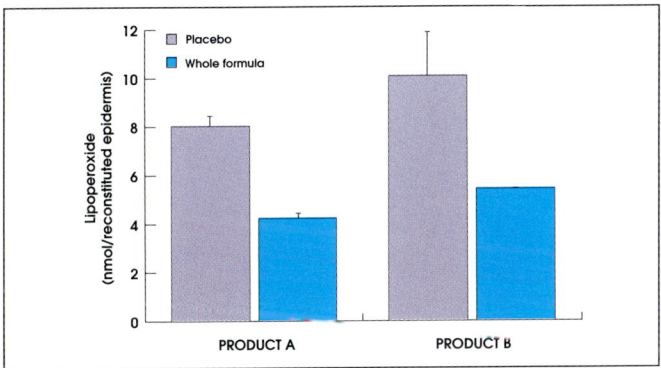

Figure 4. *Protective effect of sunscreen ingredients against UVA*

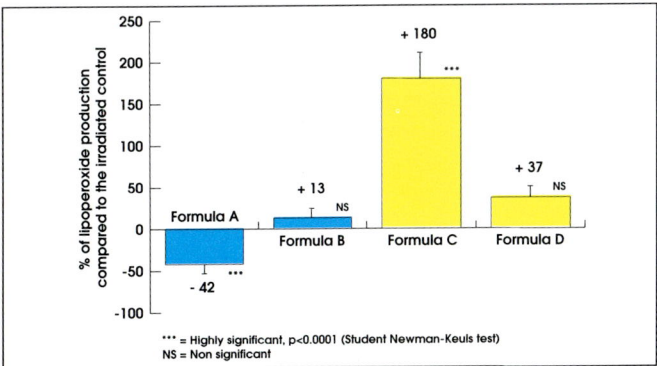

Figure 5. *Protective effect of various sunscreen formulations on UVA induced lipoperoxidation in reconstructed epidermis.*

Conclusion

In the present work, we have demonstrated that reconstructed skin or epidermis can constitute useful *in vitro* models, to study the UVA-induced epidermal damages (among which those related to oxidative stress) as well as to assess the protective potential of sunscreen ingredients.

The use of a reconstructed epidermis in the evaluation of protective effect of sunscreens against chemical phototoxicity induced by UVA

C. Cohen, R. Roguet, M. Cottin, C. Olive, J. Leclaire, A. Rougier

C. Cohen, R. Roguet, M. Cottin, C. Olive, J. Leclaire: Life Sciences, L'Oréal Advanced Research Laboratories, Aulnay-sous-Bois, France.
A. Rougier: La Roche-Posay Pharmaceutical Laboratories, Courbevoie, France.

Phototoxicity is a term used to describe all non immunologic photoinduced skin reactions.
In most case of phototoxicity, endogenous or exogenous chemical (chromophore) absorbs light and transferts the energy to, or reacts in the excited state with, cellular components.
The dissipation of energy results in an adverse phototoxic effect on the cell.
Chlorpromazine, a phenothiazine tranquilizer, was used to induce phototoxicity. This adverse reaction occurs through the absorption of the UVA radiation by Chlorpromazine metabolites.
The skin being the first organ in contact with light, tissue engineering has allowed us to reproduce *in vitro* the phototoxic response occuring at the cutaneous surface.

Materials and methods

Reconstructed human epidermis Episkin

Episkin was provided by Imedex-Saduc (Chaponost, France) as a kit containing 12 units of epidermis. One unit consists of collagen matrix (type I and III) fixed at the bottom of a plastic chamber, coated with a thin layer of collagen IV. Human adult keratinocytes seeded on this dermal substitute were grown submerged for 3 days in the medium (DMEM/HAM F12 (3:1) + 10% fetal calf serum) and exposed at the air-liquid interface for 10 days to give rise to a fully differentiated epidermis. Like the living human epidermis, Episkin presents a stratum corneum which is the ultimate state of differentiation of the epidermal cells.

UVA radiation source

The UVA source was a 1,000 W solar simulator Oriel (model 68820) presenting a 102 × 102 mm size beam. In combination with additionnal filters: Oriel n° 81050 (= Schott UG11-1mm) and Oriel n° 81019 (= Schott WG 335-3 mm) it was emitting in the 320-400 range with a maximum at 360 nm. The irradiance (13 mW/cm^2/sec) was monitored with a Osram Centra UV-meter.

Tested formulas

Two sunscreen formulas were tested for their capacity to protect the epidermis from the phototoxic reaction. Formula A contains Mexoryl®SX and titanium dioxide; formula B Mexoryl®SX – Parsol® 1789 and Eusolex® 6300 – titanium dioxide. These formulas are available from La Roche-Posay Pharmaceutical Laboratory respectively under the name of ANTHELIOS T and ANTHELIOS L. Clinical testing has been performed to determine their respective UVB and UVA protective indexes which are reported in Table I.

Table I. *Clinical protective indexes*			
	SPF1	IPD2	PPD3
Formula A	25	20	5
Formula B	60	55	12

1: Sun Protecting Factor. 2: Immediat Pigment Darkening. 3. Permanent Pigment Darkening.
Formula A: Anthelios T; Formula B: Anthelios L (La Roche-Posay Pharmaceutical Laboratories).

Treatment of the Episkin samples

100 ml of a Chlorpromazine in water dilution were applied on the Episkin surface (1 cm^2). The samples were incubated at 37° C/5% CO_2 for 24 h. Drying of the epidermis stratum corneum was achieved with a hair-drier before 2 mg/cm^2 of each sunscreen formula were applied in duplicate on the Episkin surfaces. The wells were incubated for one hour before UVA irradiation. They were rinced with PBS after irradiation and incubated overnight at 37° C/5% CO_2. The Episkin wells were then tested for cell viability using the MTT conversion test described by Mosmann (1983).

Results

Reproduction of the phototoxic reaction *in vitro*

Effect of Chlorpromazine concentration

Figure 1 describes the phototoxic phenomenon according to Chlorpromazine concentration. Chlorpromazine induced a cytotoxic reaction in Episkin with a IC50 (concentration killing 50% of the cells) of 97 nmol/Epidermal equivalent. When Episkin treated with Chlorpromazine was exposed to a UVA irradiation dose of 50 J/cm^2, the chemical treatment was much more potent in inducing cytotoxicity: IC50 dropped to 45 nmol/Epidermal equivalent.

A concentration of 50 nmol/Epidermal equivalent was selected from this Chlorpromazine dose-effect study. This concentration was effectively not cytototoxic alone, whereas in combination with 50J/cm^2 UVA irradiation it induced 50% cytotoxicity, revealing a pure chemical phototoxic effect.

UVA irradiation dose

Figure 2 describes the phototoxic phenomenon according to the UVA dose. The IC50 of UVA on Episkin was of 87 J/cm^2. In presence of Chlorpromazine (50 nmol/Epidermal equivalent) the cytotoxicity was strongly increased and IC50 reduced to 50 J/cm^2. From this study the UVA dose of 50 J/cm^2 was chosen according to its non cytotoxic effect when applied alone and to the induction of 50% cytototoxicity when given in conjonction with a non cytotoxic dose of Chlorpromazine.

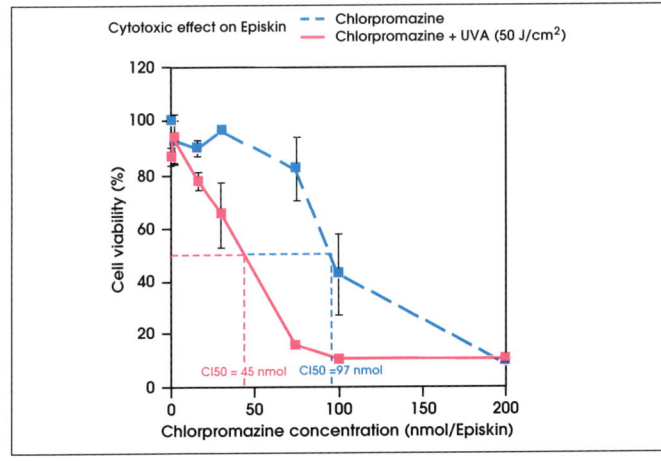

Figure 1. Phototoxic phenomenon according to chlorpromazine concentration.

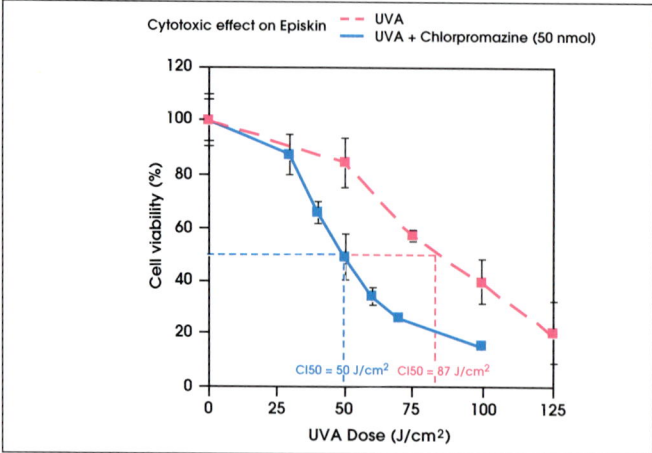

Figure 2. *Phototoxic phenomenon according to the UVA dose.*

Efficacy of sunscreen formulas against phototoxicity

Sunscreen formulas A and B were evaluated for their capacity to protect from the onset of the phototoxic reaction in comparison with their respective placebo (emulsions free of UV protective ingredients).

The UVA dose of 50 J/cm^2 induced a phototoxic reaction resulting in a decrease of 50% of cell viability when Chlorpromazine incubated Episkin wells were exposed to the solar simulator either bare or treated with 2 mg/cm^2 of placebo A or B. As shown in Figure 3, formulas A and B were totally effective in preventing from the UVA onset of phototoxic cellular damage. Thus, no difference in cytotoxicity was found when compared to non irradiated and Chlorpromazine treated (50 nmol) epidermal equivalent.

The 2 sunscreen formulas were evaluated against a 70 J/cm^2 UVA dose in an attempt to differenciate their protective potential against UVA induced chemical phototoxic reaction. As shown in Figure 4, the phototoxicity was enhanced for the irradiated Episkin control as well as placebo A and B. Formula B remained totally effective and to a lesser extent formula A was still providing a significant protection (cell viability 65%).

Discussion

The use of reconstructed epidermis has allowed us to reproduce the phototoxic reaction *(Fig.1* and *2)*. The different conditions were fulfilled so that the mechanism of phototoxicity can occur in vitro, *i.e.* the need for the drug or its metabolites to reach viable cells in the skin, the penetration of appropriate wavelength through the skin and the absorption of photons by the photosensitizing chemical.

In this study accurate results were obtained by the use of in vitro skin which presents a good reproducibility. These in vitro experiments demonstrated that chemical phototoxicity reaction was dose-dependent on drug concentration as well as UVA exposure.

The use of sunscreen formulations was also easily reproduced using this model and allowed us to assess their capacity to prevent this chemical side effect. Formula A and formula B were able to protect epidermal cell viability against phototoxicity induced by a 50 J/cm² UVA dose and a Chlorpromazine concentration of 50 nmol/Epidermal equivalent *(Fig. 3)*. When increasing the UVA dose to 70 J/cm² *(Fig. 4)*, the phototoxic reaction was intensified and a maximal protection was still provided by the Mexoryl®SX-Parsol® 1789-Eusolex® 6300-titanium dioxide formula.

Conclusion

Reconstructed skin or epidermis constitute a useful in vitro model:
→ to study the phototoxic potential of topically applied chemicals,
→ to assess the efficacy of sunscreens against this adverse reaction and especially formulations providing very high UVA protection.

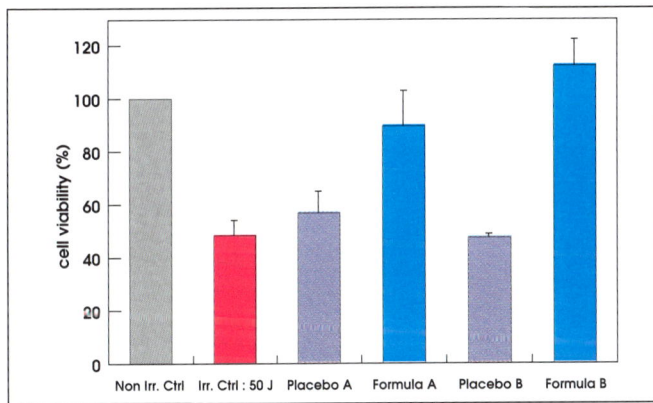

Figure 3. *Sunscreen formulas efficacy against chloropromazine phototoxicity induced by UVA (50 J/cm²).*

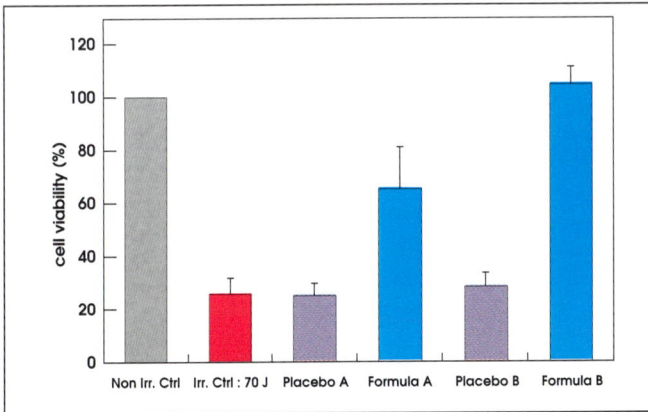

Figure 4. *Sunscreen formulas efficacy against chlorpromazine photoxicity induced by UVA (70 J/cm²).*

Prevention of solar urticaria using a broadspectrum sunscreen and determination of a solar urticaria protection factor (SUPF)

J.L. Peyron, N. Raison-Peyron, J. Meynadier, D. Moyal, A. Rougier, C. Hourseau

J.L. Peyron, N. Raison-Peyron, J. Meynadier: Department of Dermatology, Saint-Éloi Hospital, Montpellier, France.
D. Moyal, C. Hourseau: L'Oréal Applied Research and Development, Clichy, France.
A. Rougier: La Roche-Posay Pharmaceutical Laboratories, Courbevoie, France.

Solar urticaria (SU) is a rare photosensitivity disorder.
Within 5 to 10 min of sun exposure, patients experience itching, erythema, and patchy or confluent whealing. Chronically exposed skin (face, harms) is generally less susceptible to be involved than areas normally covered. All solar wavelengths can be effective for SU induction.

Antihistamines or PUVA preventive treatments remain difficult. Another alternative could be the use of sunscreen products. Unfortunately, most of them are not sufficiently effective on the whole UV range, particularly in the UVA wave band which is mainly responsible for the elicitation of SU [1-4].

The aim of the present work was to determine the solar urticaria protection factor (SUFP) of a broadspectrum sunscreen highly efficient both in the UVB and UVA wavelengths.

Materials and methods

Tests products

– ANTHELIOS L La Roche-Posay Pharmaceutical Laboratories (SPF 60, UVAPF 12*): UVB filter 5% (EUSOLEX® 6300), TIO$_2$ 5%, UVA filters 6.75% (MEXORYL® SX and PARSOL® 1789), in O/W emulsion.
* Persistent Pigment Darkening method [5].
– Vehicle (without filtering system).

Patients

10 volunteers, 5 males and 5 females aged from 21 to 73 years, with skin type 2 and 3, unexposed to the sun or solar simulator since a minimum of 3 months.
Test area: the back.

UV source

– 1000 W Xenon Arc solar simulator (Dermolum UM-W, Müller, Germany) equipped with a monochromator, the UV-output of which was monitored with a thermopile.

– Spectral bands used for irradiation:
Experiment 1   – 285-320 nm (UVB)
                    – 320-400 nm (UVA)

Experiments 2 and 3 – 310 ± 10 nm (UVB)
                    – 335 ± 10 nm (short UVA)
                    – 360 ± 10 nm (long UVA)

Clinical assessment

Clinical assessment of erythema and swelling was performed in the early minutes following each UV exposure dose.

Study design

For each experiment, the minimal urticarial dose (MUD) was determined after application of increasing doses of UVB and/or UVA.

Experiment 1

The susceptibility to SU of each patient was assessed in the UVB and in the UVA range.

Experiment 2

The minimal urticarial dose (MUD) on untreated area was determined for each patient and for each triggering spectral band.

Experiment 3

The protective effect of the sunscreen was assessed. Follow-ing the application of either 2 mg/cm^2 of the broadspectrum sunscreen or its vehicle, the MUD was determined again for each patient in each triggering spectral band defined in experiment 2.

SUPF was then determined for each patient as follow:

$$\text{SUPF} = \frac{\text{MUD with the sunscreen or its vehicle}}{\text{MUD without any product}}$$

The SUPF of the product is the arithmetical mean from all the individual SUPF found in each patient.

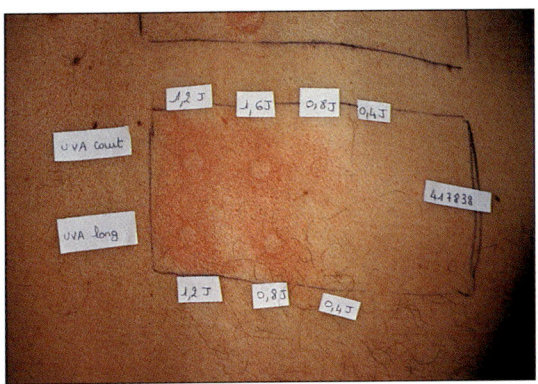

Results

Experiment 1

7 patients responded to UVA exposure (long UVA: 3, short UVA: 1, both: 3), 1 to UVB and 2 to UVB + UVA.

Experiment 2

The MUD without product ranged from 0.08 to 1 J/cm² in the long UVA, from 0.04 to 2 J/cm² in the short UVA and from 4 to 60 mJ/cm² in the UVB.

Experiment 3

The SUPFs of the vehicle were 2.7, 2 and 3.3, respectively in the long UVA, short UVA and UVB.
The SUPFs of the sunscreen were 75, 56 and 133, respectively in the long UVA, short UVA and UVB.

Conclusion

These experiments settled that solar urticaria can be elicited by the different parts of the sun UV spectrum.

	Table I. *Individual results*									
Volunteers	N° 1 BRU...	N° 2 BEV...	N° 3 MAR...	N° 4 FER...	N° 5 DOS...	N° 6 DUF...	N° 7 LAM...	N° 8 CHA...	N° 9 PAR...	N° 10 BLA...
Experiment 1 Spectral band of elicitation	UVA ------	UVA UVB	UVA ------	UVA ------	UVA ------	------ UVB	UVA ------	UVA UVB	UVA ------	UVA ------
Experiment 2 MUD										
– long UVA (J/cm^2)	1	0.5	------	0.3	1	------	0.7	0.08	0.4	0.4
– short UVA (J/cm^2)	2	0.1	1.8	------	1	------	------	0.04	0.4	------
– UVB (mJ/cm^2)	------	5	------	------	------	60	------	4	------	------
Experiment 3 MUD with sunscreen										
– long UVA (J/cm^2)	> 30	> 20	------	36	50	------	56	8	40.2	32
– short UVA (J/cm^2)	40	5.8	0.2	------	40	------	------	2	45	------
– UVB (mJ/cm^2)	------	700	------	------	------	9,600	------	400	------	------
MUD with vehicle										
– long UVA (J/cm^2)	4	1	------	0.9	2	------	2.8	0.16	0.8	1.2
– short UVA (J/cm^2)	4	0.2	3.6	------	2	------	------	0.08	0.8	------
– UVB (mJ/cm^2)	------	20	------	------	------	240	------	8	------	------
Broadspectrum sunscreen SUPF										
– long UVA	> 30	> 40	------	120	50	------	80	100	100.5	80
– short UVA	40	58	34	------	40	------	------	50	112.5	------
– UVB	140	------	------	160	------	------	100	------	------	------
Vehicle SUPF										
– long UVA	4	2	------	3	2	------	4	2	2	3
– short UVA	2	2	2	------	2	------	------	2	2	------
– UVB	4	------	------	------	4	------	2	------	------	------

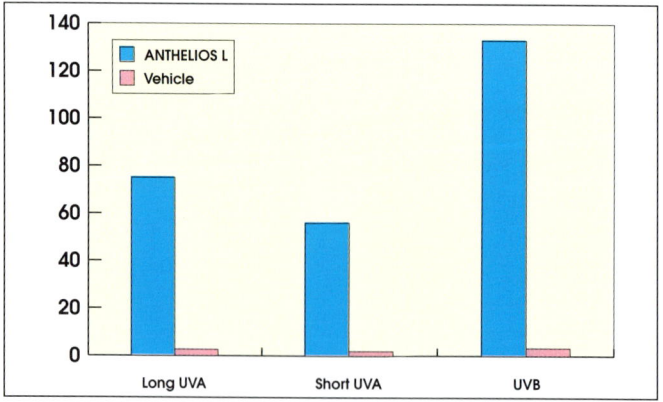

Figure 1. *Solar urticaria protection factors in each triggering spectral band (mean values).*

Moreover most of the patients reacts to very low doses of UV light, particularly in the UVA wavelengths, confirming the extreme skin sensitivity to this photodermatosis.

Our results clearly showed that the use of sunscreens can be considered as an interesting alternative in the prevention of SU. However, to be effective against urticaria induction these sunscreens must provide highly efficient filtering properties, not only in the UVB but also in the UVA part of the solar spectrum.

References

1. Harber LC, Holloway R. Immunologic and biophysical studies in solar urticaria. *J Invest Dermatol* 1963: 41: 439-43.
2. Ranits M, Armstrong RB, Harber LC. Solar urticaria: clinical features and wavelength dependence. *Arch Dermatol* 1982; 118: 228-31.
3. Leenutaphong V, Hölzle E, Plewig G. Pathogenesis and classification of solar urticaria: a new concept. *J Am Acad Dermatol* 1989: 21: 237-40.
4. Horio T. Solar urticaria. In: Lim HW, Soter NA. eds. Clinical photomedicine, New York, Marcel Dekker Inc, 1993: 181-92.
5. Chardon A, Moyal D, Hourseau C. Persistent Pigment Darkening Response as a Method for evaluation of ultraviolet. A protection assays. In "Sunscreens, Development, Evaluation and Regulatory Aspects", Marcel Dekker Inc, 1997: 559-82.

Protection of the Skin against Ultraviolet Radiations
A. Rougier, H. Schaefer, eds. John Libbey Eurotext, Paris © 1998, pp. 207-211

Pretreatment of human skin with a sunscreen or dihydroxy-acetone (DHA) prevents photoprovocation-induced polymorphous light eruption (PLE) and keratinocyte (KC) ICAM-1 expression

H. Stege, C. Ahrens, C. Billmann-Eberwein, T. Ruzicka, A. Richard, A. Rougier, J. Krutmann

H. Stege, C. Ahrens, C. Billmann-Eberwein, T. Ruzicka, J. Krutmann: Department of Dermatology, University of Dusseldorf, Germany.
A. Richard: La Roche-Posay Pharmaceutical Laboratories, 86270 La Roche-Posay, France.
A. Rougier: La Roche-Posay Pharmaceutical Laboratories, Courbevoie, France.

Polymorphous light eruption represents an abnormal response of human skin to UV radiation, especially to UVA-radiation (UVAR), which is characterized by interindividual polymorphic but intraindividual monomorphic skin lesions. In immunohistochemical studies PLE was characterized by increased and prolonged expression of proinflammatory molecules in the epidermis, such as ICAM-1 on the surface of keratinocytes (KC) [1].

Commonly used strategies to protect human skin against deleterious effects exerted by UV-radiation include topical application of sunscreen formulations as well as self-tanning ointments. In recently published studies [2], it has been demonstrated that dihydroxyacetone (DHA), which reacts with skin surface proteins in producing brown polymers, potentiates the efficacy of conventional broadspectrum sunscreens, particularly in the UVA range.

Anthelios L is a recently developed sunscreen which contains both UVB and UVA filters and thus should be suitable to prevent the induction of lesions in PLE patients. In addition, Autohelios is a DHA containing ointment which induces an ocre-brown pigmentation with poorly defined photoprotective abilities.

Purpose: Does topical application of a UVA/UVB filtering sunscreen or pretreatment with DHA prevent the induction of experimentally induced skin lesions and ICAM-1 expression in PLE patients?

Material and methods

PLE patients

n = 10, diagnosis clinically and histologically proven, unexposed to sun lignt or solar simulator irradiation for a minimum of 4 months.

Products tested

Self tanning ointment: 5% DHA in O/W emulsion (Autothelios, La Roche-Posay Laboratoire Pharmaceutique).

Sunscreen: O/W emulsion (Anthelios L, La Roche-Posay Laboratoire Pharmaceutique) containing: 5% UVB filter (Eusolex® 6300), 6.75% UVA filters (Mexoryl®SX – Parsol® 1789), 5% micronized TiO2, [SPF 60, UVAPF 12 (PPD) 55 (IPD)].

UVA protecting factors
UVAPF of the products tested were previously determined according to the Persistent Pigment Darkening methods (PPD) on 10 healthy volunteers. The UVAPF obtained were:
– DHA pretreatments   =   1.75
– Broadspectrum sunscreen =   12

Treatments

Self tanning ointment: 1 application/day (day – 4 to – 1 before UVA irradiation protocols I or II).

Sunscreen: 1 application (2 mg/cm2) 20 min before each irradiation protocols I or II.
Control: Unprotected skin area (self tanning ointment or sunscreen).

Photoprovocation protocols

UV-radiation: UVA 1 (340-400 nm); System Dr. Sellmeier 2000 device (Sellas, Ennepetal, Germany)

Protocol I: Increasing UVA-doses during 5 consecutive days (20, 20, 30, 40, 60 J/cm^2).

Protocol II: One single UVA-dos(100 J/cm^2)/day during 3 consecutive days.

End points

Clinical examination was performed by the dermatologist and signs of PLE were recorder.

Immunohistochemistry was performed on skin punch biopsies according to the labeled streptavidin-biotin method (LSAB) [3] using the ICAM-1 antibody Mab 84H10. The biopsies were taken from the untreated skin which were exposed to photoprovocation protocol II and from the Anthelios L or Autohelios treated skin areas, which were also treated with the same photoprovocation protocol (n = 5).

Results

Effect of topical application of UVA/UVB sunscreen

In 10/10 patients photoprovocation testing either with increasing UVA-doses up to 60 J/cm^2 or 1 × 100 J/cm^2 UVA on 3 consecutive days induced PLE-lesions in unprotected or untreated skin. In 9/10 patients application of the UVA/UVB protecting sunscreen Anthelios L completely prevented the induction of PLE lesions using the photoprovocation protocol I. The broadband sunscreen Anthelios L also prevented the experimental induction of PLE-lesions in 9/10 volunteers after 3 consecutive irradiations with 100 J/cm^2 UVA *(Table I)*, indicating that application of Anthelios L was effective in the prevention of the induction of PLE lesions in the same volunteers regardless of the photoprovocation protocol used. In immunohistochemical studies [photoprovocation protocol II (n = 5)] the KC ICAM-1 expression could be detected in experimentally provoked PLE-lesions, but not in sunscreen-protected skin areas *(Table II)*.

Effect of topical application of 5% DHA

In 5/8 patients pretreatment with Autohelios completely prevented the experimental induction of PLE-lesions which were provoked in all tested individuals using both protocol I and protocol II *(Table I)*. In experimentally induced PLE-lesions, increased KC ICAM-1 expression

Table I. *Prevention of experimental induction of PLE lesions after topical application of Anthelios L or pretreatment with Autohelios*

Volunteers	Untreated skin (protocol I)	Untreated skin (protocol II)	Anthelios L treated skin protocol I	Anthelios L treated skin protocol II	Autohelios pretreated skin protocol I	Autohelios pretreated skin protocol II
1	++	++	−	−	n.d.	n.d.
2	++	++	−	−	−	−
3	+++	+++	−	−	−	−
4	++	++	−	−	−	−
5	++	++	−	−	n.d.	−
6	+	++	−	−	+	+
7	+	+	−	−	+	+
8	++	++	−	−	−	−
9	++	++	−	−	−	−
10	+++	+++	++	++	+++	+++

Table II. *Prevention of experimental induction of KC ICAM-1 expression in the UVA-exposed skin of PLE patients after topical application of Anthelios L or pretreatment with Autohelios*

Volunteers	Untreated skin protocol II	Anthelios L treated skin protocol II	Autohelios pretreated skin protocol II
2	++	-	-
3	+++	-	-
4	++	-	-
8	++	-	-
9	++	-	-

+ weak ICAM-1 expression, ++ moderate ICAM-1 expression, +++ very strong ICAM-1 expression, – no ICAM-1 expression.

could be observed, whereas no KC ICAM expression could be found in DHA-pretreated and UVA-irradiated skin (photoprovocation protocol II) *(Table II)*.

Conclusion

These studies indicate that both the sunscreen and, to a lesser extent, the DHA preparation tested provide significant protection against the experimental induction of skin lesions in PLE patients. They also suggest that induction of KC ICAM-1 expression and development

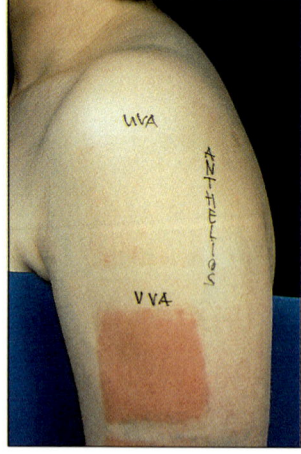

Figure 1. *You can see erythematous and papular reaction in UVA-irradiated skin area, but not in Anthelios L protected skin area.*

of skin lesions in PLE patients are closely linked and may be causally related. In previous studies, a 1 week treatment of human skin with DHA was found to induce skin pigmentation, resulting in a UVA protection factor of 1.75. It is therefore unlikely that the protective effect of DHA is due to a sunscreen effect of the DHA-induced skin pigmentation. Because UVA-radiation-induced skin lesions in PLE patients and UVA-radiation-induced KC-ICAM-1 expression previously were shown to involve the generation of reactive oxygen species, it is tempting to speculate that DHA application to human skin may have anti-oxidative consequences [4].

References

1. Norris PG, Barker JNWN, Allen MH, Leiferman KM, McDonald DM, Haskard DO, Hawk JLM. Adhesion molecule expression in polymorphic light eruption. *J Invest Dermatol* 1992; 99: 504-8.
2. Moyal D, Hourseau C, Binet O, Rougier A. Efficacy of dihydroxyacetone treatment in addition to a broadspectrum sunscreen in the prevention of polymorphous light eruption. P148 12th ICP, Vienna, Austria, Sept. 96.
3. Hsu SM, *et al.* Use of avidin-biotin-peroxidase complex (ABC) in immunoperoxidase techniques: a comparison between ABC and unlabeled antibody (PAP) procedures. *J Histochem Cytochem* 1981; 29: 577.
4. Grether-Bech S, Olaizola-Horn S, Schmitt H, Grewe M, Jahkne A, Johnson JP, Briviba K. Sies H, Krutmann J. Activation of transcription factor AP-2 mediates UVA radiation – and singlet oxygen-induced expression of the human intercellular adhesion molecule 1 gene. *Proc Natl Acad Sci USA* 1996; 93: 14586-91.

Achevé d'imprimer par Corlet, Imprimeur, S.A.
14110 Condé-sur-Noireau (France)
N° d'Imprimeur : 33152 - Dépôt légal : novembre 1998

Imprimé en U.E.